HOSPITALS IN TRANSITION
THE RESOURCE MANAGEMENT EXPERIMENT

Tim Packwood, Justin Keen and Martin Buxton

Open University Press
Milton Keynes • Philadelphia

Open University Press
Celtic Court
22 Ballmoor
Buckingham
MK18 1XW

and

1900 Frost Road, Suite 101
Bristol, PA 19007, USA

First Published 1991

British Library Cataloguing-in-Publication Data
Packwood, T.
   Hospitals in transition: The resource management experiment. - (State of health series)
   I. Title II. Keen, J. III. Buxton, M.
   IV. Series
   362.10941
   ISBN 0-335-09951-3
   ISBN 0-335-09950-5 (pbk)

Library of Congress Cataloguing number is available.

Printed in Great Britain

HOSPITALS IN TRANSITION

CONTENTS

	Acknowledgements	vii
	Series Editor's Preface	ix
	Introduction	1
	Why this book?	1
	Structure of the book	2
1	**RM in Context**	5
	Introduction	5
	National issues	5
	The origins of RM	11
	National experiment to national policy	20
	Effects of the NHS Review	25
	Major local influences	27
	Conclusion	30
2	**Project Planning and Management**	31
	Introduction	31
	Local RM policies	31
	Project management	34
	Project planning	36
	Conclusion	40
3	**The Implementation of RM**	41
	Introduction	41
	Information and information systems	41
	Organisation and structure	56
	Organisation development	70
	The nature of RM implementation	73
	Conclusion	78
4	**The RM Process**	79
	Introduction	79
	The nature of the process	80
	RM at the individual level	84
	RM at the sub-unit level	90
	RM at the unit level	98
	Linkages between levels	104
	Adoption of the RM process	106
	Conclusion	110

5	**The Resource Requirements of RM**	111
	Introduction	111
	RM implementation	116
	RM processes	120
	Conclusion	127

6	**Benefits of RM**	129
	Introduction	129
	The overall performance of the six sites	130
	Service production benefits	132
	Service activity benefits	134
	Patient outcomes	137
	Perceptions of consultants and nurses	138
	Perceptions of key managers	142
	Conclusion	143

7	**Conclusions and Implications**	144
	RM and its evaluation	144
	Major conclusions	145
	Lessons from the RM Initiative	150
	The balance of evidence	157

Reflection	**The Organisation Transformed**	163
	Introduction	163
	Collaboration, authority and control	163
	The external environment	168

Appendix 1	**Methodology and Methods**	170
	Commissioning of the research	170
	Research methods	171

Appendix 2	**Time Series Performance Data for the Six Sites**	178

Glossary		186

References		189

ACKNOWLEDGEMENTS

Over the course of any large and lengthy study, researchers depend on the time and goodwill of many people. We have been fortunate in the general support and encouragement we have received. One of our greatest debts is to staff in the six sites, with whom we worked for two and a half years. It was not always easy to make appointments or obtain the data we wanted, but the courtesy and helpfulness of the vast majority of staff rarely faltered and they afforded us remarkable access to their work.

Where it is necessary to the understanding of the data, and where direct comparison is helpful, data and examples have been attributed to particular sites. Where the precise origin of data is not important and examples and quotations are used illustratively, the sources are anonymised.

Our Advisory Group helped us to steer through sometimes difficult waters, and, like candid friends, alerted us when we were in danger of going off course. We are thus grateful for the help in a personal capacity of: Mr M. Garner, Mrs J. Griffin, Dr C. Ham, Mr J.N. Johnson, Ms A. Kauder, Professor M. Lahiff, Mr R. Nicholls, Dr H. Sanderson and Mr T. Scott. Dr Ham also provided us with helpful steerage in another persona, as Editor of the series of which this book is the first-born.

Rebecca Malby was commissioned by us for a short period to undertake a study of the role of nurses in RM. We are very grateful for her commitment and the clarity of thought she brought to this area of our work.

The technical side of the production of this book has involved a number of people. Richard Baggaley and Sue Hadden of Open University Press were always helpful, and a pleasure to deal with.

Stuart Neilson made a decisive contribution towards the end of the study, with his advice on producing camera-ready copy.

Finally, another great debt is owed to Nicky Gillard who as well as preparing this manuscript, has coped with our demands during the whole period of the study. She has, crucially, remained calm, which is more than we can say for ourselves.

This study depends to a significant extent on qualitative data. While many people have shared their views and experiences of Resource Management with us, and we have striven to reflect accurately the experiences of the sites (and taken on board many of their comments and those of our Advisory Group on earlier versions of this text), the assessments made here are ours, and we take full responsibility for them. They should not be ascribed to the Department of Health, or any of the six sites.

TP, JK, and MB

SERIES EDITOR'S PREFACE

Health services in many developed countries have come under critical scrutiny in recent years. In part this is because of increasing expenditure, much of it funded from public sources, and the pressure this has put on governments seeking to control public spending. Also important has been the perception that resources allocated to health services are not always deployed in an optimal fashion. Thus at a time when the scope for increasing expenditure is extremely limited, there is a need to search for ways of using existing budgets more efficiently. A further concern has been the desire to ensure access to health care of various groups on an equitable basis. In some countries this has been linked to a wish to enhance patient choice and to make service providers more responsive to patients as 'consumers'.

Underlying these specific concerns are a number of more fundamental developments which have a significant bearing on the performance of health services. Three are worth highlighting. First, there are demographic changes, including the ageing population and the decline in the proportion of the population of working age. These changes will both increase the demand for health care and at the same time limit the ability of health services to respond to this demand.

Second, advances in medical science will also give rise to new demands within the health services. These advances cover a range of possibilities, including innovations in surgery, drug therapy, screening and diagnosis. The pace of innovation is likely to quicken as the end of the century approaches, with significant implications for the funding and provision of services.

Third, public expectations of health services are rising as those who use services demand higher standards of care. In part, this is stimulated by developments within the health service, including the availability of new technology. More fundamentally, it stems from the emergence of a more educated and informed population, in which people are accustomed to being treated as consumers rather than patients.

Against this background, policy makers in a number of countries are reviewing the future of health services. Those countries which have traditionally relied on a market in health care are making greater use of regulation and planning. Equally, those countries which have traditionally relied on regulation and planning are moving towards a more competitive approach. In no country is there complete satisfaction with existing methods of financing and delivery, and everywhere there is a search for new policy instruments.

The aim of this series is to contribute to debate about the future of health services through an analysis of major issues in health policy. These issues have been chosen because they are both of current interest and of enduring importance. The series is intended to be accessible to students and informed lay readers as well as to specialists working in this field. The aim is to go beyond a textbook approach to health policy analysis and to encourage authors to move debate about their issue forward. In this sense, each book presents a summary of current research and thinking, and an exploration of future policy directions.

Dr Chris Ham
Fellow in Health Policy and Management
King's Fund College

INTRODUCTION

WHY THIS BOOK?

The Resource Management (RM) Initiative in the NHS was formally announced in 1986. Its purpose was:

> to enable the National Health Service to give a better service to its patients, by helping clinicians and other managers to make better informed judgements about how the resources they control can be used to the maximum effect (DHSS, 1986a).

It was to be undertaken as a national experiment in six acute hospitals which would serve as pilots. It was also stated that the experiment would be 'objectively evaluated'.

The Health Economics Research Group (HERG) at Brunel University, directed by Martin Buxton, indicated interest in evaluating the costs and benefits of RM at the pilot sites. In 1988 HERG was commissioned by the Department of Health and Social Security (DHSS) to undertake a three year evaluation of the RM experiment. An interim report on the development of RM was presented to the DHSS in mid-1989 and the final report was submitted to the Department in January 1991.

Although by no means obvious in 1986, RM represents an enormous cultural change for the operation of the NHS. The extent of this change has inevitably been overshadowed by the more radical changes resulting from the NHS Review of 1989, which accepted the value of RM and proposed its extension across the service.

Because RM is going to be an important part of health service management, now and in the future, it seemed right to attempt to place an account of its nature and an assessment of its implications, costs and benefits, strengths and weaknesses, before as large an audience as possible, as rapidly as possible. But the authors were conscious that this audience was, in all likelihood, a number of potential audiences with rather separate interests in RM. One audience was certainly the NHS, concerned to learn from the experiment how best to introduce RM and get it working. The members of this audience would, of course, be seeking rather different answers according to the nature of their engagement with RM: whether they were involved as service providers or general managers; whether they worked at regional, district, unit or sub-unit level; whether they had responsibilities for implementing some aspect of RM or were having to live with the results, and so on. A second potential audience was offered by those who are interested in the way in which health policies, or public policies in general are implemented and converted into process. The RM Initiative was an example of a national policy that had to be applied at the periphery of a decentralised and professionalised service, and which was, as is so often urged upon governments by policy analysts, explicitly experimental. From this standpoint, RM represented an interesting test case for social scientists. A third, if smaller and probably more critical, audience was constituted by those interested in the mechanics of evaluating policy initiatives. The methodology adopted by HERG and the experience of its application might prove of use to other researchers engaged, or wishing to engage, in a related exercise.

In writing for the interests of such a divergent group of possible readers, the authors have concentrated on providing an evaluation of the RM experiment, in the six pilot hospitals, drawing heavily upon the research report that was presented to the Department of Health. But an attempt has been made to set RM within the context of current health policies and to reflect more generally upon its character as a policy initiative.

STRUCTURE OF THE BOOK

It follows from what was said above that the concern is principally with evaluating the RM Initiative as a whole but to do so means describing and analysing the experiences of individual sites. The sites concerned are:

Arrowe Park (now Wirral) Hospital, Wirral HA
Freeman Hospital, Newcastle HA
Guy's Hospital, Lewisham and North Southwark HA
Huddersfield Royal Infirmary, Huddersfield HA
Pilgrim Hospital, South Lincolnshire HA
Royal Hampshire County Hospital, Winchester HA

The multi-faceted nature of RM, and the different emphases and rates of progress made at the sites, mean that some topics lend themselves to treatment in general terms and others require fairly detailed comments on developments at individual sites. Details are attributed to specific named sites when it is important to understand specific differences in approach and experience. In other cases examples from the sites are used illustratively without specific attribution. In addition, direct but anonymised quotations are used throughout the text to illustrate most vividly some of the opinions expressed to the researchers. These quotations should not be taken as attempts to summarise 'average' opinion. Throughout the book extensive use is made of boxed tables and diagrams to illustrate, explain and support points made in the text, and a Glossary, explaining the major technical terms and initials used, is provided at the end of the book.

It should be stressed that the report makes no attempt to describe the overall experience of any one of the sites: this has to some extent been done elsewhere, in articles and on video (e.g. Chantler, 1989; Department of Health 1989a, 1989b). Neither does the book provide a blueprint for the implementation and operation of RM, although some of the key lessons learned from the sites are drawn out in Chapter 7, and practitioners may draw lessons relevant to their own interests from elsewhere in the text. The methodology of the study is explained in Appendix 1. This might be usefully read first by those whose main interest is in the mode of evaluation.

The structure of the book is set out below, together with some suggestions as to which material is likely to be directly relevant to a particular audience without necessarily working chronologically through the text.

- *Chapter 1, RM in Context*, discusses the policy developments which preceded and accompanied the RM Initiative, including the NHS Review, briefly reviews the origins and history of RM itself and indicates the major local influences affecting the individual sites during the course of the Initiative (policy analysts).

- *Chapter 2, Project Planning and Management*, presents the objectives for RM set by the sites themselves, and discusses their approach to project planning and management. The six sites adopted different approaches in implementing some aspects of RM, and these differences are highlighted (RM project leaders, policy analysts).

- *Chapter 3, The Implementation of RM*, concentrates on some of the finer detail about the implementation of RM, dealing with the computerised information systems, organisation and structure and organisation development (RM project leaders, NHS practitioners).

- *Chapter 4, The RM Process*, makes a change of emphasis, towards analysis of the nature and impact of RM as a management process. The key characteristics of this process at different levels of the organisation are described and evidence of the presence of the RM process drawn, using illustrative examples, from across the sites (RM project leaders, NHS general managers and service providers).

- *Chapter 5, The Resource Requirements of RM*, presents, by site, the additional costs of implementing RM, and discusses the resource implications of the RM process within the sites (RM project leaders, NHS general managers and service providers, policy analysts).

■ *Chapter 6, Benefits of RM*, discusses the service benefits associated with RM and the perceptions of key participants at the sites (RM project leaders, NHS general managers and service providers, policy analysts).

■ *Chapter 7, Conclusions and Implications*, summarises the main points made in the earlier chapters; drawing out some of the key lessons for other sites embarking on RM, for similar national policy initiatives in the future and for policy evaluation. The chapter concludes with an assessment of the balance of evidence regarding the success of the RM Initiative. (This chapter effectively provides a summary of the key points and major conclusions of the book as a whole).

■ *Reflection, The Organisation Transformed*, turns to the future role of RM, where it has become an integral part of management processes, and offers a vision of how RM might transform hospital management (policy analysts, NHS general managers).

■ *Appendix 1, Methodology and Methods* (researchers and policy analysts).

■ *Appendix 2, Time Series Performance Data for the Six Sites* (policy analysts).

■ *Glossary* of terms used.

■ *References*.

Chapter 1

RM IN CONTEXT

INTRODUCTION

In evaluating the way in which the RM Initiative has worked, account has to be taken as factors that influence the process and product, although they are not an actual part of the RM strategy. The RM experiment could not be conducted in a laboratory and isolated from contamination by what was going on around. Indeed because it is concerned with the way in which service providers, individually and collectively, plan, manage, deliver and evaluate services for patients, successful RM has to be sensitive and responsive to other demands and pressures. A further complexity is that both the RM Initiative and the context in which it operated were dynamic, extending across the second half of the 1980s decade. During this time national and local policies and circumstances changed, as did national and local approaches to RM.

The chapter commences by briefly reviewing the major issues affecting the health services nationally in the 1980's issues which could be expected to impact upon the central operation of the RM Initiative and its application in all the sites.

The national context provides a framework for first examining the origins and initial objectives of RM, and second, for tracing its development as a national experiment. This displayed an important shift over the period of evaluation in response to the proposals for reorganising the provision of health services contained within the NHS Review (Secretaries of State, 1989a). It is hard to imagine a more dramatic change in the immediate environment of an experiment involving social institutions than that represented by the NHS Review, so some attention is given to its effects on the RM Initiative.

Finally, the focus is shifted to local contexts. Local policies and circumstances, themselves often a reaction to national concerns, inevitably influenced the application of RM in the six sites. Space does not allow an anthropological exploration of local cultures over the period of the experiment, but attention is drawn to some of the most important local factors.

NATIONAL ISSUES

In no way could the 1980s be seen as a comfortable decade for public health services. It opened with a major structural reorganisation, completed in 1982, that abolished one level of organisation, the health area, and pushed authority for providing hospital and community services down to the smaller territorial dimension of the health district. The decade closed with a fundamental philosophical reorganisation, intended to be implemented by 1991, that separated the accountability for providing and paying for health services and sought to strengthen the freedom and competitiveness of service providers. The same principles were to be applied to care in the community, where yet another attempt was made to clarify service responsibilities (Secretaries of State, 1989b).

En route there was a major initiative to improve the management of the NHS, requiring yet a further reorganisation, that was commenced in 1984 (Griffiths, 1983), and another to reshape the nature of primary care, implemented after difficult negotiations in 1990 (Secretaries of State, 1987). As the decade progressed, health services, and particularly their shortcomings, increasingly occupied the attention of both the media and the politicians.

Part of the necessity for continuously rethinking the organisation of health services came from their having to satisfy three rather different purposes. First there was the curative function, extended by medical knowledge and fuelled by public demand, that required specialised expertise and technology, and was typified by treatment in hospitals. Increased application of technology increased costs and both factors operated to reduce hospital beds. Over the decade the average number of acute hospital beds in England fell from 146,000 to 121,000 and the average length of stay for acute medical and surgical cases fell from 9.6 to 7.1 (Department of Health, 1990a). Demand increased, and despite considerable progress in developing treatments that could be applied on an out-patient or day patient basis, and specific financial targeting, by 1990 waiting lists for in-patient treatments stood at the highest level, over 900,000, since the NHS had been created. Second, there was the caring function, extended by medical success in delaying mortality and by the increased numbers of the very elderly, that required generalist expertise and facilities to alleviate the effects of ill-health, and was typified by arrangements for care in the community. The elderly, mentally ill, mentally handicapped and young disabled, who could all be categorised as chronically ill, represented national priorities throughout the 80s, but it proved hard to redistribute resources away from acute treatment. It also proved hard to develop coherent policies between the numerous disciplines and agencies involved in promoting services outside hospitals, and community care continued to rely heavily on informal carers. Third, there was the preventative function, extended by education and public campaigns, that required individual commitment and coordination between public and private agencies, and was typified by individuals being exhorted to care for their own bodies. The emphasis here has been on health promotion, with problems arising in respect of the cost effectiveness of screening programmes and wider regulatory strategies that posed dilemmas for individual and economic freedom. Prevention, it might be suggested, only represents a priority to cure where no cure exists; a situation that was apparent in respect of AIDS, which became the subject of a government containment campaign from 1986.

The three functions shared two common properties. First they evoked apparently limitless need and, second, raised questions as to the effectiveness of traditional medical care and the balance between resources expended and benefits produced. The labour intensive nature of the health service, particularly as represented by prestigious and influential professional bodies, fuelled inflationary pressures. So, too, did the 'technological imperative' (Fuchs, 1974), which led health providers to constantly seek to improve and develop their services, and the associated rise in public expectations. Throughout the 1980s the NHS demonstrated a healthy ability to consume increasing sums; total central government expenditure on health in the United Kingdom rising over the decade from nearly £12 billion to £24.7 billion, an increase in real terms of nearly 20 per cent (HM Treasury, 1991). Doubtless health has fared somewhat better than many other areas of social expenditure, but it, too, has been the subject of a deliberate and sustained effort to contain costs (Eyles, 1987). Cash limits were introduced by the Labour Government in 1976 and have subsequently been extended to the majority of the total budget. Since 1985 health authorities have been expected to make efficiency savings from their existing budgets, although cost improvement programmes have proved uncertain and imprecise (IHSM/NAHA, 1989). And paradoxically there was always a considerable element of uncertainty with regard to central funding. This can be seen in respect of the proportion of pay awards that exceeded the government's inflation forecasts that would eventually be funded centrally. Additional funding was provided for particular problems that gained political prominence, such as the AIDS epidemic, or the plight of inner London health districts, which, as part of the Resources Allocation Strategy were receiving a lower proportion of development monies than districts in regions elsewhere, which were reckoned to be more deprived of health facilities. Additional monies also came in connection with particular initiatives such as the reduction of waiting lists or RM itself.

Shortages of funds have been manifest in recurrent cash crises, marked by ward closures, curtailment of services and growth of waiting lists. Perhaps less obviously they have also been reflected in the curtailment of new building schemes and delay in the maintenance of existing plant. The NHS has also been slow in adopting the modern commercial infra-structure of computerised control and information systems.

The problems mentioned above were manifested in a series of tensions, arguably making their solution all the harder.

First, there was the tension between policy needs as seen by central government on the one hand, and by the periphery (district authorities, district and unit managers, doctors and nurses providing services directly to the public) on the other. A dilemma, according to Klein 'as old as the NHS itself' (Klein, 1989), Ham suggests that at the beginning of the decade the centre was attempting to become less involved in the running of the NHS but changed tack in 1981, with a move to increasing central control (Ham, 1986) as a means, principally, of securing efficiency. This was typified by the introduction of annual accountability reviews between levels in the service, by stricter manpower controls, by the national adoption of the Griffiths recommendations in 1984, and the requirement that health authorities undertake competitive tendering for some of the hospital support services.   None the less it remained the case that despite the presence of central views of needs, and the attempts to improve local accountability and review mechanisms, decisions regarding the application of resources to needs remained local decisions, in the hands of the professionals, local managers and the members of the local health authorities.

A second long standing tension was that between the professional service providers and the service managers. Alford's analysis, although originally applied to the American scene, is familiar here (Alford, 1975), defining professional monopolists, particularly the doctors, as 'the dominant interest', and the corporate rationalisers, particularly the managers, as 'the challenging interest'. The 1980s have seen 'the challenging interest' grow stronger, shifting from management through professional agreement in the 1982 structure, to the introduction of general managers and stronger commercial principles following the Griffiths recommendations in 1984, to the routine involvement of the professional service providers in managing their own activities and use of resources as part of RM.   The professional monopolists have been directly challenged by the government, notably in the creation of a new contract for GPs and in implementing the recommendations of the NHS Review.   Their own unity is also threatened by the functional divergencies in health services mentioned above.   The interests of a hospital consultant or intensive therapy unit (ITU) nurse are not necessarily promoted by an expansion in community care.

The third area of tension is that between service supporters (the taxpayers represented by the politicians), the service givers (those who work in the health service and directly provide or support patient treatment and care), and the service recipients (the patients).   Although surveys suggest that taxpayers do not resent funding the NHS and would indeed be prepared to pay more, the political will has been to reduce central taxation as a burden on both the economy and individual initiative.   Politicians have also attempted to strengthen the power of service recipients, emphasising that recipients are consumers and that as they are also the financers they should expect an efficiently run service and value for their money. Yet it remains a basic characteristic of health services in the United Kingdom that needs are defined by the service givers and that service supporters cannot readily act as service recipients, far less as consumers in the market place. A supporter is, more or less, perceived as healthy, whereas a recipient is, more or less, perceived as ill. The properties and behaviour attached to the two conditions remain very different. Over the 1980s the terms of exchange between the three interests have moved to strengthen political interests, ostensibly acting on the supporters' behalf. Service interests have been dented but not crushed. The government appears to have some mistrust of the expert, particularly when collectively organised, but as far as health is concerned this distrust is not necessarily widely perceived or shared by the public. The interests of the patient remains individualised, dependent and weak.

The NHS Review

The Review, published as a White Paper in early 1989 (Secretaries of State, 1989a), and to a lesser extent the new GP contract of 1990, the Griffiths Review of community care (Griffiths, 1988) and subsequent White Paper (Secretaries of State, 1989b), can be seen as both the culmination of, and as an attempt to resolve, the divergencies and tensions of the past ten years.

The Review itself commenced in early 1988 as an immediate reaction to the well publicised problems of underfunding in the NHS. It was undertaken by a committee of ministers and advisers connected with the Conservative Party and was chaired by the Prime Minister. The White Paper, *Working for Patients* which reported its recommendations was, in the event, concerned with principles of organisation and management rather than finance and was particularly concerned with the acute services. The argument of the White Paper was that both patient and staff satisfaction could be improved by reorganising the health service so that it was more competitive and cost effective. This was to be attained in three ways.

First, a separation was made between financing and providing health services. The State's responsibility for the former would remain unchanged. Provision, however, could be pluralist: by both public and private institutions. But if the State was distancing itself from the direct provision of health services, it could not withdraw from the responsibility of ensuring that standards remained satisfactory. This was to be achieved by improved mechanisms for regulation, such as compulsory medical audit and the extension of the remit of the Audit Commission.

Second, the organisation was to be improved by giving greater weight to market forces, through the introduction of managed competition. District health authorities, and those GPs who wished to do so and met the necessary criteria in terms of size of practice, would purchase health care for their population/patients by placing contracts with provider units - the hospitals or community health services. Authority and accountability could now be achieved by the contracts between purchasers and providers, rather than by relying on managerial hierarchies. Contracts could be used to secure both value for money and quality assurance. Former barriers to the market such as territorial boundaries, bureaucracy, representation and professional power were all to be reduced. Thus money could now move with the patient across health authority boundaries to gain the best terms of contract from a provider. The more work a provider unit contracted for, the more money it would receive. Decision-making and control of resources were to be delegated to the providing units that now had a financial incentive to meet local needs. Providing units could, given satisfactory management and involvement in management by their senior professionals, gain greater independence of action by withdrawing from district accountability and becoming self-governing NHS Trusts, accountable to the Secretaries of State. Authorities would be expected to operate on commercial principles, there was an end to automatic representation by local government or by the health service professionals. As regards the latter, management was to have a stronger voice in determining terms of contract and rewards.

Third, the organisation was to be improved by stronger management. At the central level the Department of Health, separated since 1988 from Social Security, was to attempt more definitively to separate its own policy making and executive responsibilities; a separation that was to be made manifest by locating the latter at Leeds! At the local level general managers and senior officers were to be members of authorities. Management was strengthened in its relationship to the professionals, and there was generally an emphasis on managing clinical activity. Local managers were given more authority to determine conditions of work, including involvement in consultant appointments, deciding consultant merit awards and in drawing up and managing consultant contracts. The latter includes ensuring that job descriptions covered responsibilities for quality of work, use of resources and extent of services provided. But the professionals were also encouraged and/or obliged to manage their own activities, as through RM and medical audit. Indeed the White Paper affirmed the value of RM. If stronger and wider management was to be a reality, better information was a necessity. One particular weakness was the limited ability to link information about treatment activities to the costs incurred. This was to be addressed by extending and accelerating the RM Initiative:

> to provide a complete picture of the resources used in treating hospital patients.

As part of this process the RM Initiative was to be extended to 260 acute units by March 1992.

The proposals elevated the health service to the forefront of political debate, although successively and rapidly to be replaced by the Community Charge, the state of education, the crisis in the Arabian Gulf and the Conservative leadership crisis. Because the Review proposals were general in nature and the product of 'armchair' or 'cabinet table' theorising rather than any trial, commentators were free to pursue their particular prejudices. Professional interest expressed fears that the former beneficent approach, providing services according to need, would be replaced by reciprocity, providing services according to the reward, and that the NHS might deteriorate from a universal service available to all, to a residual service only available to those unable to afford anything better. Professionals and various local community interests were concerned with the possibility of hospitals opting out of their districts accountability and becoming self-governing trusts. Conversely many service managers appeared to welcome the opportunities provided for stronger management, for increased freedom of action and flexibility in meeting needs.

The proposals also placed a burden on the NHS in that they imposed a tight timetable. A framework for medical audit was to be in place and the new contractual arrangements in operation by 1991. Health authorities were to be reconstituted from summer 1990, while the RM roll-out and the separation of central policy and executive functions were to begin at once. And it was not just that new structures and processes had to be put in place, health service staff had to consider new possibilities and began to work in new, and no doubt often unexpected ways. The National Health Service and Community Care Act legalising these changes received the Royal Assent on 29 June 1990.

THE ORIGINS OF RM

As defined at the beginning of the experiment in 1986 (DHSS, 1986a), the overriding aim of RM was:

> to enable the National Health Service to give a better service to its patients by helping clinicians and other managers to make better informed judgements about how the resources they control can be used to the maximum effect.

This statement indicates four key and inter-related elements contained within RM (Packwood *et al.*, 1990).

- *Improved quality of care* as a result of the service providers, the doctors, nurses and paramedics who directly treat and care for patients, having access to information about the effectiveness of different patterns of treatment and greater authority to determine the deployment of their resources.

■ *Involvement in management by the service providers* whose decisions directly commit resources to patient treatment and care. These staff have a good idea of patient need and have to ensure that this is heard in planning resource use. They are also in the best position to ensure resources are used to best effect.

■ *Improved information* to identify how resources are being used, with what effect and what are the alternatives.

■ *Stronger control of resources* that results from rational and responsible management and use of information, for resource allocation and determining service activities.

All four elements can be related back to issues of national policy which were discussed in the previous section. They were also, to a greater or lesser extent, all matters of current concern.

■ *Improved quality of care* reflected the 'technological imperative' to improve performance, rising public expectations and the existence of doubts as to the effectiveness of some forms of treatment. The medical profession had already begun to flirt with the idea of establishing formal audit procedures (Social Services Committee, 1989).

■ *Involvement in management by the service providers* reflected long standing problems of professional accountability and divergent interests between practitioners and managers. Attempts to make service providers take greater responsibility for managing resources characterised the history of the NHS (Ham and Hunter, 1988). But since 1983 and the Griffiths recommendations, doctors' clinical freedom in deciding how to apply resources to treating their patients had to reach some form of rapprochement with general management. Some hospitals had already moved to give service providers, and particularly doctors, a greater managerial involvement through creating clinical directorates at sub-unit level based on service specialties.

■ *Improved information* was necessary for more efficient and effective management. 1986 saw the first indication of a clear national policy for information technology (IT) in the NHS with the creation of a National Strategic Framework (DHSS, 1986b). Also the growing availability and improvement of computer technology made the rapid provision and manipulation of information a feasible, if expensive proposition.

■ *Stronger control of resources* was necessary to bring the NHS into line with government policies for the public sector and the economy. This was promised by developments in specialty costing and Management Budgeting (Perrin, 1988), and in case mix classification and costing (Bardsley *et al.*, 1987) that made it possible to relate the processes involved in providing individual patient treatment and care to the resource inputs. This would then make it possible to manage activities rather than resource allocation.

Cumulatively the four elements addressed by RM potentially effect all aspects of the way in which the NHS operates, which accounts for the enormous cultural change ultimately represented by RM. The combination had been foreshadowed by the Griffiths Report (Griffiths, 1983), certainly the grandparent of RM, but the means and will for their realisation were not then available. Even in 1986 few beyond visionaries and champions would have recognised the potential, or indeed the existence, of the different elements, for the statement in which they are contained was no more than a restatement of the aims of Management Budgeting given in 1985 (DHSS, 1985). To understand the origins of RM, then, means looking to Management Budgeting (MB) as an immediate parent.

Management Budgeting

MB was also an experiment, partially funded by the DHSS, to improve cost effectiveness and efficient use of resources in the health service by making the service providers aware of the costs they incurred, and getting them to take some accountability for their allocation and expenditure. The experiment commenced in four acute and two community sites in 1983 and in 1985 was extended to a further fourteen acute sites.

The first MB experiments were associated with the Griffiths Inquiry into NHS Management (Griffiths, 1983). They had been considered urgent enough by Griffiths and the DHSS to be set up as a part of, rather than as a result of, the Inquiry. Their purpose was to demonstrate how it was possible to:

> ensure that each Unit develops management budgets, which involve clinicians and relate work-load and service objectives to financial and manpower allocations, so as to sharpen up the questioning of overhead costs.

But the idea was yet older. Iden Wickings and his colleagues had experimented with the idea of clinical budgets based upon planning agreements in the 1970s (Coles *et al.*, 1974, 1976). And the possibility of producing costs in terms of clinical specialties had been recommended by the Körner Committee (DHSS, 1982-84) as providing:

the essential first step towards patient or treatment related output costing (RM Directorate, 1989).

Box 1.1 depicts something of the extended ancestry of RM.

In 1985 the Director of Financial Management on the new Management Board of the NHS, Ian Mills, undertook a review of the progress being made with MB. In general he was disappointed. MB had:

so far, not generally been seen as making any worthwhile contribution to the planning and costing of patient care (DHSS, 1986a).

Although sites had established a good technical foundation for MB, they had been less successful in making it part of a management system (DHSS, 1986a). Perhaps given the understandable desire to show quick results, attention had been focused on improving the information base rather than on spending time in clarifying the management arrangements. Crucially, MB was not linked in to planning processes (Pollitt *et al.*, 1988). This question of emphasis was also to continually occupy RM. But there were other flaws in MB. First, it was experienced as a finance dominated strategy. The information systems lacked the capacity to relate cost data to clinical activities in a sufficiently sensitive way to encourage service providers to review their activities. The motivation for many clinicians was to use information to provide better patient care and cost data aggregated by specialties was of little use. A second, and related problem, was that MB proved a 'top-down' strategy. It was driven from unit or even district level. It hardly encouraged collaboration, either between service providers and general managers or between the service providers, themselves. Managers supplied the service providers with information and discussed its implications with them, rather than service providers supplying managers with information and feeding it into the planning process. As a consequence the service providers had no sense of owning the information and viewed it with distrust, and their engagement with MB appeared to have little overall effect.

Not all involved with MB gave critical assessments. It had prepared the way for RM in establishing data collection mechanisms and getting service providers and managers to think of the relationship between resources and activities. As later with RM, many felt that the evaluation had come too soon, and in their joint statement, the Joint Consultants Committee (JCC) and Management Board accepted that the MB experiment had:

coincided with a period of considerable organisational uncertainty (DHSS, 1986a).

Box 1.1   The origins of RM

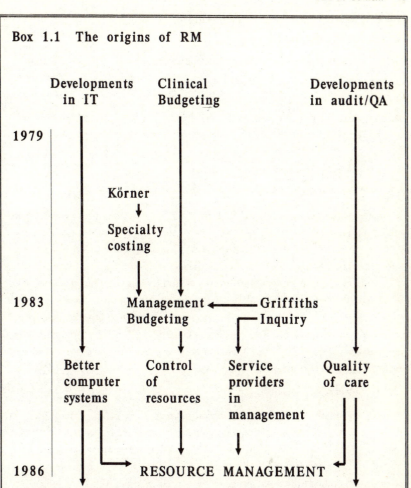

So in 1986 RM emerged as a final attempt to recast MB to overcome the problems listed above:

we are determined to establish once and for all, as objectively as possible, the practicality or otherwise of developing cost-effective information services for clinicians in our acute units (DHSS, 1986a).

MB in the two community sites had been judged to be more successful. This was not to be recast but rather rolled-out, as RM, to a further fifteen second generation sites.

Resource Management

The objectives initially defined for RM are listed in Box 1.2. Leaving aside the familiar difficulties in deciding whether improvements occur in patient care, the subsidiary objectives are also difficult to identify unambiguously. One man's waste is another's economy and one woman's beneficial discussion is another's wasted time. Judgements as to success or failure were bound to be difficult to reach and heavily qualitative and subjective. The Notice setting up the experiment suggested that if RM was to be judged successful, local managers, doctors and nurses needed to be able to answer the questions listed in Box 1.3, confidently in the affirmative. But these questions, too, were primarily qualitative and subjective in nature and raised issues of definition and measurement.

At the outset it was felt necessary to distance the new approach from MB:

bearing in mind the rather narrow, financially exclusive, meaning associated with this term [Management Budgeting] by large numbers of doctors, both the Management Board and the JCC (Joint Consultants Committee) consider it would be sensible in future to refer to the search for better information systems for clinicians and nurses as 'resource management' (DHSS, 1986a).

It was consistent with what had been learned from the experience of MB that RM was to be a joint venture promoted by the Management Board, the JCC and local management. Initially it was to involve four acute sites, Freeman, Guy's, Huddersfield and the Royal Hampshire, that were already beginning to think about some aspects of what subsequently became RM, although they differed considerably in their respective emphases. By 1986 the number had been increased to six. The experience with MB can be seen in the pre-requisites required of the sites:

■ doctors and nurses must already play a senior management role;

■ agreement to introduce case mix planning and costing;

Box 1.2   Objectives of RM

Principal objective

Introduction of a new approach to resource management and to demonstrating whether or not this results in measurable improvements in patient care.

Subsidiary objective

Provision, for clinicians, of information which enables them to:

1.   Identify areas of waste and inefficiency.

2.   Benefit from clinical group discussion and review.

3.   Highlight areas which could benefit from more resources.

4.   Identify and expose the health care consequences of given financial policies and constraints.

5.   Understand the comparative costs of future health care options and hold informed debates about such options.

Box 1.3   Tests for the success of RM

1. Has the management scheme involved fully the clinicians?

2. Has this enabled the clinicians to have a positive influence on the management of resources of the unit?

3. Have the information systems provided data relevant to patient care and has the information been of value to clinicians in providing that care?

4. What have been the direct and indirect costs of implementing the scheme and have these costs been justified by the resulting benefits of the scheme?

5. Has the time-input required by clinicians to implement the scheme been considered by the clinicians themselves to be beneficial to patient care?

■ application of management development and training programmes.

Statements of the key aims referred to:

■ medical and nursing 'ownership' of the system, developing management processes and information systems that would meet their requirements;

■ the application by service providers of comparative data on resource use for both monitoring clinical performance and determining deployment of resources;

■ producing accurate basic patient activity data.

In addition to meeting the pre-requisites and being in agreement with the aims mentioned above, the six initial sites were chosen to represent a balance between teaching (Freeman and Guy's) and non-teaching and provide a wide geographic spread. In terms of size they varied from Arrowe Park with 850 beds to the Royal Hampshire with 460 and, on a different dimension, from Guy's with 3,000 staff to Huddersfield with 1,500. They also represented different experience in respect to MB: three, Clatterbridge, Freeman and Huddersfield were second generation sites and a fourth, Guy's, had been involved with the early clinical budgeting experiments. Freeman and Guy's had both assisted in the Griffiths Inquiry, and two of the six, Guy's and the Royal Hampshire, had already adopted strong sub-unit organisational structures based on clinical directorates. All six were at different stages in developing the information systems necessary to support RM. A further part of the strategy, then, was that through their diversity the six hospitals selected to participate in the experiment would be able to act as reference sites for the rest of the service. They would act a 'test bed', feeding back information on the strengths and weaknesses of hardware and software, of desirable structures and the need for management development and training. As Ian Mills expressed it:

> we do not want to be too prescriptive about which model or parts of models districts will want. We hope to end up with a limited shopping list - perhaps five or six total scenarios with a greater number of individual modules - but there is, as yet, no ideal or fixed solution (quoted in Millar, 1987).

But acting as laboratories for RM would come to represent a heavy, and sometimes unwelcome, burden for the sites.

The final point to record regarding the origins of RM in the six sites was that two hospitals, Arrowe Park and Clatterbridge, were located in the same health authority, Wirral. At the outset they both encountered problems of funding. As a result RM at Arrowe Park did not get under way until 1987 and Clatterbridge withdrew from the experiment altogether. It was replaced in 1988 by Pilgrim Hospital in South Lincolnshire, which had also been a second generation MB site and had begun to develop computer systems to support specialty and individual consultant budgeting.

RM was never, however, inclusive to the six experimental sites. Other hospitals across the nation pursued their own versions of RM and some of these came to be seen as leaders in the field. In at least one case, at the Radcliffe Infirmary, Oxford, an evaluation of RM was undertaken (Oxford Regional Health Authority, 1988).

NATIONAL EXPERIMENT TO NATIONAL POLICY

It is significant that throughout its life as a national experiment, and beyond, RM has received a high profile from the Department of Health. Those staff centrally responsible for the initiative, and they have always been few in number, have seen the need to work at motivating the service. They have been publicly visible stumping the country 'preaching the message' to professional audiences, contributing articles to professional journals, producing a series of information sheets reporting on progress with RM and more substantial reports on different aspects of the initiative (RM Directorate, 1989; NHS Resource Management Unit, 1990).

RM was congruent with developments in other areas of government, such as the Financial Management Initiative (FMI) within the civil service, in locating accountability for the use of resources where these were committed. At a later stage it could be seen as instrumental to the wider and more fundamental changes proposed in the NHS Review. Second, RM as a policy was very much the product of central government, following on as described earlier, from the Management Budgeting Experiment in 1986. Ian Mills had played a major role in getting RM started, although it was created as a joint venture, subject to joint evaluation, between the Management Board, the JCC and local management in the experimental sites (DHSS, 1986a). Mills, who was seconded to the Department of Health from the private sector, acted as a catalyst in getting the experimental sites to develop some common view of the ends, if not the means, to be expected from RM. He proved a doughty and committed champion of RM. So much so that when his period of secondment as Director of Financial Management ended in 1988, he retained responsibility for RM on a part time basis, and as a separate directorate, until he finally left the NHS in June 1989.

The departure of Ian Mills and the resumption of responsibility by the Directorate of Financial Management, under the leadership of Sheila Masters, coincided with an apparent change in the central approach to RM. Before 1989 it is possible to see the Department of Health treating RM as a discrete experiment. After the NHS

Review was published in January 1989 elements of RM, such as the need to involve doctors in management and provide improved activity and cost information, were treated as self-evident truths requiring general application; while from April 1989, RM itself had become an approved policy to be rolled-out across the NHS. In other words, after 1989 Department policy carried the message that the experiment was over and the new Director inherited a programme whereby RM would systematically become part and parcel of the normal ethos for all acute hospitals. This change of tack, represented in diagram form in Box 1.4, was seen as 'premature' by many involved with RM in the local sites. It was severely criticised as a breach of faith by the medical professional bodies supposedly sharing in the evaluation of RM with the NHS Management Board (CCSC, 1989) and later, by the National Association of Community Health Councils (ACHCEW, 1990).

The roots of this disagreement lie in the origins of RM as a joint initiative between the Management Board and the medical profession, and in the question of what constitutes an evaluation. When the experiment was first announced in 1986 it was stated that a provisional evaluation of likely success would be undertaken in 1988 and that if this were favourable, RM would be implemented in other acute units over 1988-92. The joint statement on RM by the JCC and the NHS Management Board also said that once the initial development and implementation period was complete, RM:

> will be objectively evaluated before any final decisions are taken about what is right or appropriate for the NHS as a whole (DHSS, 1986a).

The RM Directorate undertook an interim evaluation in Autumn 1988 (RM Directorate, 1989) concluding that it was:

> too early to judge probable achievement levels. Most of the sites have not fully implemented their plans and the Resource Management approach is not yet therefore fully operational.

But that:

> a significant momentum is building up as the potential benefits come into clearer focus.

It had taken longer than had been first thought to get RM 'off the ground'. But Ian Mills was clear that time was required at the beginning for sorting out the issues and problems. The definition and scope of RM had to emerge through practice.

The JCC and Central Consultants and Specialists Committee (CCSC) also produced a brief assessment of progress at the same time (RM Directorate, 1989), reporting that:

Box 1.4   Central policy towards RM

1986

1987   HN(86)34 announcing RM   RM as a
             Initiative (November)   discrete
                                                       national
                                                       experiment

1988

1989   RM Directorate/JCC/CCSC
             interim evaluation (October)

             NHS Review (January)   RM as
             First roll-out sites (March)   national
             HERG interim report (July)   policy
             CCSC final evaluation (October)

1990

1991
             HERG final report (February)

the clinicians in each district remain optimistic, though ultimately uncommitted about the benefits of Resource Management.

Given that progress had not been so rapid as had been hoped in 1986, the detailed evaluation to measure the impact on service quality and the costs of the new organisational and information arrangements, was to be undertaken in October 1989. By now the Health Economics Research Group (HERG) at Brunel University had been commissioned by the DHSS to undertake an external evaluation of the costs and benefits of RM (see Appendix 1). In their interim report, published in July 1989, the authors concluded:

that in none of the six sites is RM to be found across the whole hospital.

And that:

most of the change to date has been predicated on expectations of benefit rather than evidence (Buxton *et al.*, 1989).

The CCSC (1989) produced their own evaluation and concluded that:

whilst encouraged by the experience of the experimental sites, the CCSC is not yet convinced that the evidence so far justifies extending the RM Initiative to additional sites.

No comprehensive summary of the 1989 evaluation exercise has yet been produced by the RM Directorate, thus giving credence to the idea that the Department of Health had ceased to treat RM as an experiment.

A distinction between the pre- and post-1989 approaches can also be seen in the mechanisms by which the Department worked with the six sites. Pre 1989 emphasis was placed on the local Project Steering Committees in each site and on the national Chairmens' Project Steering Committee. The former, chaired by a senior figure from the district or hospital concerned who was committed to RM, formulated the local strategy and reviewed progress. Its membership was partly functional, including the local project manager and staff involved in implementing different aspects of RM, and partly representative, including clinicians and nurses who would be required to apply RM, regional officers and generally the Director or Deputy Director of the central RM Directorate. The committee thus provided a link between the different interests involved with RM and, in particular, provided a means for the Centre to learn what was actually happening on the ground and to promote the policy. The national Chairmens' Committee brought the Chairmen and Project Managers from each of the six sites together with staff from the central RM Directorate. It was chaired by the Director or his deputy and provided a forum for reviewing collective progress, identifying particular needs and considering the impact of national policy on the RM experiment.

After 1989 the Chairmens' meetings were run down. The six sites were still asked to send representatives to national meetings arranged by the central Directorate but these were likely to be focused on particular issues, rather than general progress, and their membership was not necessarily restricted to the experimental sites. The Financial Management Directorate, of which the RM Directorate once again formed part, had many other demands to meet in connection with the Review proposals. Regions had been given a leading part in the roll-out of RM across the NHS, and members of the central team were obliged to give more of their time and support to the new Regional RM Co-ordinators. Local site Project Steering Committees continued to meet, if fitfully, and the RM Directorate tried to ensure that one of its staff attended. The message that came across was that the Department of Health wanted to work closely with innovators and committed local management in a number of fields. And although the six sites were certainly at the leading edge of NHS development by virtue of their involvement with RM, and would probably continue in this position for the foreseeable future, innovation was neither exclusive to the six sites or to RM.

Staff in the local sites were aware that the relationship with the centre had changed. To some this occasioned relief, they could get out of 'the goldfish bowl' and get on with providing health services. Another reaction was one of inevitability. The RM experiment had finished; it had provided a catalyst for change but now it was time to move on to other things. Others expressed uncertainty. Different aspects of RM were still being developed, there was no 'tested package' that could be widely adopted. And the environment and objectives of the post-Review NHS appeared very different from those applying when RM was launched in 1986, yet somehow the experiment had now become the accepted standard. At the same time RM appeared to have become incorporated within the larger consequences of the NHS Review. The Department of Health were well aware of the latter fear. Reassurance was given to the service and Sheila Masters wrote in the professional press (Masters, 1990) stating that:

> the RM Initiative is not inextricably linked to any of the other proposals in the White Paper.

None the less many participants in our research saw the NHS Review and its implementation as changing the nature of RM and in particular as changing the ground rules of the experiment.

RM is history.

UGM

RM has not been run as a proper experiment. It has been assumed by government to be a success.

Consultant

EFFECTS OF THE NHS REVIEW

Because RM is an explicit part of the strategy proposed in the Review and because its principles and elements are felt to underpin and/or strengthen many other parts of the strategy, attitudes of some staff towards RM became subsumed within wider political attitudes to the government's health service policy. Those who supported this policy supported RM, those who opposed the policy were drawn to oppose or express scepticism towards RM. But it was striking that some, including many clinicians, remained supportive of RM while expressing opposition to other aspects of the Review (Keen, 1990).

The reverse side of this coin is that inclusion in the Review gave RM some force. The government obviously meant business and part of this business was RM. This attracted support, or acceptance, for RM from those who were impatient for change to occur or who saw it as unavoidable. It was also seen by some of our respondents as supplying impetus and drive to the implementation of RM, as a means of realising some of the benefits proposed in the Review. It certainly appeared to give a greater emphasis to the application of computer systems.

The Review has certainly been seen as dominating all local agendas. The local sites saw attention diverted from RM, to grapple with such issues as self-government or contracting, before RM itself could in any sense be thought of as complete. And, in many cases, it was the attention of key individuals for RM, such as general managers and financial and information staff, who were already in short supply, (Black *et al.*, 1989; Committee of Public Accounts, 1990) whose efforts were diverted. The sites saw Review requirements as shifting attention to collect new data and develop new working processes from those required by RM. Some respondents saw this as positive, part of a new learning curve. Others referred to a sense of duplication; of similar data being requested, of another set of change strategies being implemented, of yet another project management plan being devised, to serve the various proposals.

Certain topics covered in the Review appear to be particularly relevant to RM.

■ *Contracting.* Some staff felt that contracting implied a relationship of reticence between purchaser and provider which was the opposite to the open flow and analysis of data which was the hallmark of RM. Contracting thus fuelled sensitivities about the movement of data from unit to district. District staff tended to argue for access to activity and costing data in that it helped both in constructing contracts and in managing their operation in terms of volume and quality. Unit staff were more likely to be resistant to the movement of data, fearing that it might place them at a disadvantage in the contracting process. Arguments then arose as to which level 'owned' the RM data and were exacerbated where the information technology was the result of substantial district investment and development of RM. Similar sensitivities existed within units regarding data relating to individual activities passing to specialty or unit level, and that relating to specialties passing to unit. In that the Review proposals emphasised the unit as the focus for operational management, some clinicians became increasingly cautious regarding access to, and distribution of, 'their data', and the issue of safeguards to access became more prominent.

Similarly, contracting fuelled sensitivities between the various levels in respect of the accuracy of data. Lower levels exhibited a reluctance to release or accept data from higher levels which they felt to be inaccurate or open to misinterpretation. Some clinicians were reluctant to participate in coding on these grounds.

Finally, work on developing contracts exacerbated fears that particular forms of data were being emphasised, particularly cost data, and that the cost control element of RM was being emphasised at the expense of service quality. To those of this mind, the RM experiment was a decoy to impose tighter financial management upon the service providers.

To a certain extent this idea [RM] is excellent because we need to know how much everything costs. But I fear that it is being used as a tool to show we can provide more care with less resources.

Staff Nurse

An emphasis on costing represented a particular difficulty for the six experimental sites which to some extent had played down the costing element of RM as a deliberate policy.

But again the reverse of the coin was that RM paved the way for the Review proposals, and those who actually had to grapple with the task of developing service specifications and prospectuses, usually the general and financial managers, became markedly more appreciative of RM as a means of constructing realistic and informed contracts. Some units welcomed the wider distribution of data as a means of challenging the financial allocations adopted by higher authorities. Similarly some consultants were at pains to make information about their work available in order to demonstrate their efficiency.

■ *Quality*. The emphasis in the Review on promoting and maintaining quality emphasised the quality of care aspect of RM. Monitoring of service provision and resource utilisation is, as suggested in Chapter 4, a crucial stage in the RM process. In particular the requirement for medical audit worked to facilitate RM; giving additional point to the collection of activity data and requiring the service providers to familiarise themselves with this data and to collaborate between themselves.

■ *Organisation*. Here the Review proposals appeared to strengthen the move, apparently inherent in RM, towards some form of sub-unit organisation, focused on specialty groupings, as a major management structure for service provision. Such groupings also provided an appropriate framework for medical audit and could usefully act as the agents for unit management in the contractual process.

MAJOR LOCAL INFLUENCES

Examples of local factors that were perceived in the six sites as influencing RM are briefly discussed below. Some of these applied throughout the period of the experiment, others at particular stages. Inevitably effects were felt more keenly in some parts of the hospitals, and by some individuals, than others.

To help relate these factors to the sites concerned and give at the outset some sense of the scale of their work, Box 1.5, taken from performance data supplied by the sites (and set out in more detail in Appendix 2) indicates revenue budgets and selected activity data for 1988-89, the commencement of the HERG evaluation.

■ *Site mergers*. In 1986, when the RM experiment commenced, it included two hospitals from Wirral District Health Authority (DHA), Arrowe Park which had only been opened as a DGH in 1982, and the older Clatterbridge Hospital. Clatterbridge subsequently withdrew from the experiment but in 1989 the decision was made to merge the two hospitals to form the Wirral Hospital. When Arrowe Park had originally opened it had to integrate staff from a number of smaller hospitals that had been closed, each with their own traditions and ways of working. Now there was the same need for integration between the two larger hospitals. In its RM strategy Arrowe Park placed considerable emphasis on the

Box 1.5 Activity and budgets for the six RM hospital sites, 1988-89

	Arrowe Park	Freeman	Guy's	Huddersfield Royal Infirmary	Pilgrim	Royal Hampshire County
Revenue budget £ million	30.0	40.0	59.0	22.3	16.6	21.1
In-patient episodes						
with day cases	40,599	38,513	37,170	25,303	27,010	21,114
without day cases	34,300	29,714	34,295	23,860	24,125	19,073
Length of stay - days	6.9	6.8	7.02	5.2	7.0	8.0
Turnover interval - days	1.8	2.5	1.30	2.0	3.1	1.8
Out-patients						
referrals	39,745	24,557	63,433	33,480	21,573	20,436
consultant initiated	145,633	95,463	250,997	119,527	60,895	66,174
Available bed days	299,884	258,962	303,705	180,156	243,520	168,788

directorate structure and it was decided to merge the two sites within common directorates, rationalising accommodation and services between the sites as necessary.

■ *Site expansion.* Builders are a continual presence in large acute hospitals, but two of the six sites, Guy's and the Royal Hampshire hospitals, were in the middle of very large programmes of capital development. At the Royal Hampshire, in particular, this presented problems for service planning, requiring attention from general managers and obliging directorates to forecast future needs and demands. However the presence of a directorate structure did appear to be successful in reminding service providers of impending changes and keeping their implications in mind when considering current plans.

■ *Financial problems.* The necessity of finding a better way of managing a dramatic budget reduction provided the trigger for Guy's to move to the directorate structure which foreshadowed RM (Smith and Chantler, 1987; Chantler, 1989). Freeman hospital was also in part motivated to introduce RM by the expectation of being in a better position to argue the case for financial recognition of a heavy out of district workload. At one point or another during the course of the project Arrowe Park, Guy's, Pilgrim and the Royal Hampshire hospital all faced problems of overspending on their annual revenue budgets.

> You must remember that the RM project is being severely hampered by financial cutbacks. Thus I have one ward closed, beds dissipated over the hospital site, cancelled theatre sessions, potential shortage of nurses.
>
> Consultant

Such problems have provided a challenge to RM and the role it has played in responding to such crises is discussed in Chapter 6. The existence of financial problems has certainly been a cause of criticism for RM, and has made it more difficult to convince sceptics that the expenditure was justified.

■ *Seeking Trust status.* The decision as to whether or not to apply for Trust status and the preparation of the application generated a great deal of debate, and was seen by many of the participants in our research as detracting from RM. This was certainly the view expressed by the five senior consultants, one from each of the pilot sites apart from Guy's, who wrote to the Secretaries of State in March 1989, suggesting that RM could satisfy the major intentions of the NHS Review and that consideration of self government was a diversion of energy. But this was a highly sensitive issue. Some staff at the sites were concerned that this letter misinterpreted their position. Freeman Hospital, for example, formally withdrew from the opinions expressed and clarified their position with the Secretaries of State.

Involvement in the RM experiment meant that the six sites were seen as occupying the forefront of hospital development, so there was wide interest and speculation in the press regarding their intentions.

In the event three, Arrowe Park, Freeman and Guy's, eventually requested to become responsible for their own management as NHS Trusts in the first round of applications. In all three cases the decision to apply was championed by senior managers and the presence of RM was advanced as a positive factor. In all three cases some staff and community interests doubted the wisdom of the decision, and in the case of Guy's, it was attended by public controversy among the service providers. All three applications proved successful. But the issue also took up some time and energy and stimulated debate in the other three hospitals that decided against an early application.

■ *Other priorities*. Although receiving priority in terms of the development of RM, all six hospitals were part of districts that had to satisfy other priorities. In every case districts had priorities in terms of the development of those community-based services for the chronically ill that represented national service priorities. The districts that contained Arrowe Park, Freeman and Pilgrim hospitals also held priorities for the up-grading of other hospital facilities. Competing local demands were accepted as inevitable but also as inevitably restricting what RM could accomplish within the time available for the experiment.

CONCLUSION

RM addresses a number of long standing problems in the NHS. Although in many ways it can now be seen as 'embryonic' within the Griffiths recommendations for managing the NHS, neither the means nor climate for achieving its objectives were present in 1983. Even by 1986, when more of the pre-requisites for success were available, the introduction of RM represented a tremendous change for the NHS. But the period since 1986 during which RM has been implemented has seen a major change in context following the NHS Review. This has markedly increased the turbulence in the environment with which RM has had to cope. In the process it has ceased to represent the dominant concern in the experimental sites, and because of the early roll-out the sites, themselves, now share their role in the development of RM.

Chapter 2

PROJECT PLANNING AND MANAGEMENT

INTRODUCTION

When the RM Initiative was announced in November 1986, the six sites did not have a blueprint showing them how to proceed. RM was a collection of ideas drawn from experiences with and perceptions of earlier initiatives, including Management Budgeting, and the task of the sites was both to meld the ideas into a coherent whole and then implement them. It was thus akin to a Research and Development project, and much of the early work at the sites had a strong R and D flavour. Yet there was also considerable pressure on the sites to succeed in implementing RM, with the Department of Health, in particular, needing to find 'a better way' of managing hospitals.

In this chapter, the approaches developed by the sites to the planning and management of the implementation of RM are discussed. Chapter 3 then outlines the progress made by the sites in implementing the different elements of RM, and reflects on the nature of the implementation process.

LOCAL RM POLICIES

Although all of the six sites accepted the national objectives of RM as defined in Health Notice (86)34 (DHSS, 1986a), they also had their own statements of objectives which reflected their preoccupations and the way in which they were approaching RM. Statements of the local objectives are set out in Box 2.1, together with a note of their apparent emphases. Some of the sites presented their objectives differently in different contexts, and as the local experiment evolved, so too did the details of local objectives. Nevertheless, the principal stated objectives remained broadly constant over the course of the study.

In fact, inspection of Box 2.1 shows common themes occurring between the sites. In the case of seeking improved cost-effectiveness and clinical involvement in management these represent obvious and general objectives of RM. The emphasis on de-centralisation as against improved clinical and managerial relationships can be explained by the organisational structure adopted by the particular hospital, and it is clear that even before the NHS Review there was some feeling that new ways of working were required to manage increasing demands on hospital resources.

Box 2.1   Local objectives of RM

Emphases

Arrowe Park
Locally the project was seen as a way of bringing in
external assistance and funds to assist in breaking
into a spiral of increasing throughput combined with
static revenue. From the DHA's point of view there
was the additional opportunity of integrating the new
RM system at all three units (in the District) with
other major initiatives being undertaken - particularly
the investment in Information Technology.
(Project Plan, as published in RM Directorate, 1989)

Improved
cost-effectiveness

District interest

Freeman
To develop the culture, organisation and technical
infrastructure to enable managers in all disciplines to
plan and control their services in accordance with
mutually acceptable objectives. In particular to know
the financial consequences of workload to enable senior
medical, nursing and management staff to plan for the
consequences of technological change, tertiary referrals
and an ageing population during a period in which
limited growth would enable the development of a limited
number of services only.
(Project Plan, as published in RM Directorate, 1989)

Stronger management

New demands

Guy's
To introduce de-centralised management by combining the
clinical responsibility of doctors with managerial
responsibility for resources. This will achieve:
1. Greater efficacy, with more resources freed for patient
   care.
2. More responsive management that is closer to the clinical
   services provided for patients.
3. Day to day management delegated to the clinical team
   with improved quality of decision making.
4. Improved operational performance and environment for
   both in-patient and out-patients.
(Project Plan, as published in RM Directorate, 1989)

Decentralisation

Clinicians as managers

Huddersfield
To provide management with the correct tools.
To involve clinicians in management through:
1. Discussions on problems and priorities within the Unit.
2. A monthly review process of resource use and clinical
   activities.
A subsidiary but necessary condition for these is the
collection of accurate and timely data.
(Huddersfield RM Report, 1988 - unpublished document)

Stronger management

Clinicians as managers

Better information

Box 2.1 (continued)

Emphases

Pilgrim
1. To collect significant clinical data for use by doctors in order to investigate protocols and consider outcomes. The ability to look at cases in large volume is advantageous in this.
2. To encourage doctors to enter into budgetary discussion with management.
3. To manipulate nurse management data in order to identify how to use nursing resources more effectively.
4. Generally, to plan nurse staffing needs on an informed basis.
5. To capture information in order for management to understand clinical activity and its cost, and consequently to enter into a dialogue with doctors.
6. To help clinicians appreciate the cost of resources they command and to look for cost effectiveness, where this is consistent with clinical practice.
(Project Plan, as published in RM Directorate, 1989)

Improved quality of care

Improved relationships between general managers

Improved cost-effectiveness

Royal Hampshire
The primary aim of RM in the Royal Hampshire County Hospital is to provide the eight directors of Clinical Services with the information necessary to plan and manage the services they provide effectively and efficiently within predetermined budgets. An important further extension of this is to utilise that information that must be available to achieve the primary aim in order to:
1. Plan services corporately over a longer timescale.
2. Unlock traditional patterns of resource allocation.
3. Re-align both services and resources to meet changing health needs.
(Royal Hampshire, RM Plan 1988/89 - unpublished document)

Decentralisation

Improved cost-effectiveness

Corporate planning

New demands

PROJECT MANAGEMENT

At the start of the RM Initiative, each site had to submit an outline project plan to the Department of Health, both as an exercise in clarifying objectives and strategies and as a basis for funding bids. For the most part, these documents were very general in nature, outlining a range of things that had to be done and setting broad objectives, most of them closely in line with the objectives stated in HN(86)34. That these first plans made general statements about RM is consistent with its early status as an R and D project. (Box 2.2 lists some of the lessons that sites felt they would learn as a result of taking part in the Initiative). But of greater interest here is the nature and quality of the project planning process thereafter, as the sites started to implement RM and developed their understanding of its nature.

The sites came early to the view that the implementation of RM comprised both discrete projects separate from the on-going activity of the hospital, and organisation-wide developments. Of particular interest here were the projects, which displayed a number of features common to the six sites. Each had a project manager and an identifiable project team for most or all of the period of the study. The project team comprised members of hospital staff and typically also district staff and representatives of companies involved in designing and implementing computer systems. The project teams were concerned at different stages with most aspects of RM, but their principal efforts were focused on two areas: implementation of new computer systems and the organisation and delivery of training courses, seminars and other events where RM-related issues were discussed.

Each site had a steering committee, which provided a forum for formal links with the Department of Health. Within the sites, the composition of both steering committees and project teams varied, though in general authoritative figures including the UGM, key consultants and the Director of Nursing Services (DNS) were members of both.

Some elements of RM implementation were handled as sub-projects: notably, each site had a nursing project team. One or more nurses were seconded to the RM project, including a designated project nurse, whose principal tasks were to implement ward-based computer systems and co-ordinate training in the use of the systems. The project nurse - and often also the DNS or a senior nurse - were members of the main project teams. In some cases they were involved in all discussions about RM, in others their presence was largely symbolic, and nursing development was essentially separate from the rest of RM.

The project planning and management tasks were thus largely the province of the project manager and team. Organisation development, in contrast, involved both the project team and staff in the wider organisation. Between them, they had to initiate

Box 2.2   RM as an R and D project: what would be learned

	Domain	*Knowledge*
1.	Organisation structures	Which ones 'work': how to involve consultants and nurses formally in management processes
2.	Information technology	How to design and implement a 'case mix database', linked to operational systems
3.	Information	Clinical coding; patient costing; budgeting; patient classification
4.	Change	How to effect major organisational change in hospitals
5.	RM	How the elements fit together

change, manage it and continuously evaluate the emerging roles and relationships. Box 2.3 illustrates the relationships at different stages of the project planning process. This emphasises that the project manager and members of the project team were involved in both types of change process.

For both projects and organisation-wide developments, the project manager and team members required the authority to execute the projects satisfactorily and on time. The fact of involvement in the Initiative legitimised the setting up of project teams, and seems initially to have persuaded some people to become members. Some of the project managers also had line management posts, and attended key unit level meetings in the latter capacity.

But on an operational level, project managers in general lacked the authority they felt was needed to effect the changes they were charged with making. Authority was often, though not always, in practice retained by unit and district officers; and compounding the problem, the scale and breadth of RM meant that project managers simply lacked the time to both tackle operational tasks and formally manage the project. To counter this, project managers and many team members demonstrated considerable energy and drive, and for at least some developments had the enthusiastic backing of general managers and other key figures, and this enabled them to make progress with implementing the many aspects of RM.

PROJECT PLANNING

Project planning processes at the sites were analysed according to the four dimensions identified by Henderson and Venkatraman (1989), and to a fifth that was found to be relevant to RM:

■ completeness, the extent to which all the necessary elements have been included;

■ comprehensiveness, concerning the level of detail required for planning;

■ consistency, which is the extent to which the different elements of the plan fit together;

■ validity, the degree to which the planning process is a correct one for an organisation;

■ flexibility, the extent to which planning responds to external and internal changes, in particular growing understanding of the nature of change processes.

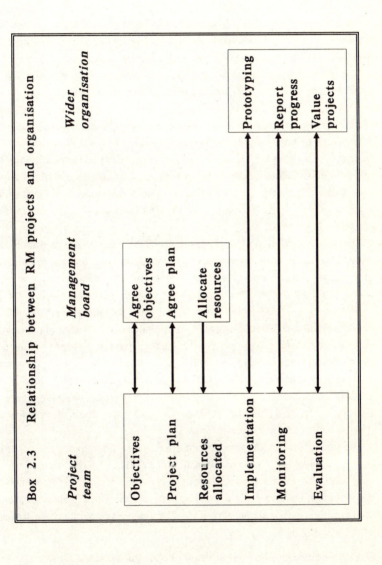

Box 2.3   Relationship between RM projects and organisation

Project team	Management board	Wider organisation
Objectives	Agree objectives	
Project plan	Agree plan	
Resources allocated	Allocate resources	
Implementation		Prototyping
Monitoring		Report progress
Evaluation		Value projects

■ *Completeness.* The sites' written project plans for 1988-89 and 1989-90 all devote a great deal of space to the development of central RM databases, ward nursing systems, costing and coding. These elements represent the common core of the plans. The desire to implement RM across the hospitals was always recognised, but the main focus at the sites was the in-patient systems. Latterly, sites have been extending into out-patients, though in general this work was still at the development stage by the end of the study.

The sites differed in their emphasis on training and on organisation development. Evidence on training both from written plans and interviews suggests that sites ranged from a highly structured approach at the Royal Hampshire and Arrowe Park to a deliberately *ad hoc* approach at Freeman. Approaches to organisation development were similarly varied, at least in the early stages, with some sites tending to view it as essentially unpredictable, and others as in significant measure amenable to planning. By the end of the project a consensus was emerging around the view that certain aspects of development could be planned and others could not, though there was still disagreement as to where the balance lay.

The sites also differed in the extent to which they focused on information and on information technology strategies. In general, the early focus at the sites was on designing and implementing the technology, on the grounds that the need for a 'case mix database' was one of the 'givens' of the experiment. As a result, the sites' strategies tended to be technology driven: the initial emphasis was on collecting data (on in-patients) which was already being collected in operational information systems. Sites in general modified their approaches in this area during the course of the Initiative, and began to consider their information needs in more detail, particularly in relation to the provision of reports to different levels of the organisation, and began work on the design of out-patient systems. However, even by the end of the study period the main focus of cross-hospital developments remained on in-patients.

The sites' plans for RM focused almost exclusively on implementation, rather than on the identification and realisation of benefits. Indeed, such significant statements about benefits as were written were associated with the operational hospital information systems at Arrowe Park and the Royal Hampshire, rather than for more central elements of RM. The absence of such plans for RM as a whole was striking.

■ *Comprehensiveness.* The level of detail of planning increased considerably over the period of the study, this detail being manifested in two ways. For the computer systems developments, and in some sites for training also, there were increasingly detailed written plans, culminating in bulky specification documents and implementation timetables. These obviously required a great deal of thought and discussion resulting in a detailed end product, and were produced by all sites.

Organisation development required all staff closely involved in implementing RM to think through the consequences of their various strategies and activities. The result here was an understanding of how RM would change organisation structures and processes. All of the sites increased in the depth and sophistication of their thinking in this area as they progressed.

Even by the end of the study, however, there were differences in views between sites as to the level of detail required for planning, particularly in respect of organisation development. Some took the view that detail was crucial, and produced detailed plans for all aspects of RM, whereas others felt that it was more important to leave room for manoeuvre as RM developed, and so used their plans as frameworks within which to manage.

■ *Consistency*. The extent to which the different elements of RM were planned so as to fit together again increased over time. This, perhaps, was the area which most emphasised the experimental nature of RM: the sites were given the task of working out how the elements fitted, so as to make a whole. Sites started with different conceptions of what RM was about, some broad, others more narrowly focused. Over time those with narrower visions broadened them, so that there was eventually a large measure of agreement at the sites about the general nature of RM: the similarities between the sites greatly outweighed the differences.

By the end of 1990 the sites had progressed to the point where it was reasonably clear how the main elements of RM and its supporting infrastructure fitted together: organisation structures were clarified to the point where sites could identify where further work was required on organisation development, and sites were working towards identifying who needed what kind of routine reports. These informed the planning and timetabling of activities for getting the complete RM process in place.

One test of the consistency of project planning is the extent to which sub-projects were included in overall plans. The nursing projects were felt by many to be an important element of RM, and typically had their own, often very detailed, project plans. However, the extent to which these plans were integrated with overall project plans varied greatly, some being closely related and others being developed largely in isolation from the main projects. Thus while there was consistency at a general level between the elements of RM, there were still instances of their not being integrated into overall plans.

■ *Validity*. Whether or not the plans for RM suited the sites' broader objectives is difficult to comment upon here, but the evolutionary nature of RM and its need to involve a wide range of staff suggests that it must be closely related to the culture of the organisation. This point is highlighted by major perturbations such as *Working for Patients*, which changed the environment for all of the sites, and hence changed the place of RM within the hospitals.

What is striking, however, is the extent to which the RM project plans were developed in isolation from the sites' annual planning cycles. The isolation was not total, with the implementation of RM acknowledged as an important task in annual plans, but there was little evidence that RM would be used to address particular issues. Rather, RM was perceived to be of very general value in improving services.

- *Flexibility*. As noted in Chapter 1, the sites were subjected to a number of national and local influences. Moreover, there were developments within the hospitals, principal among which was a growing understanding of the scale of the implementation among those most closely involved. All of the sites tended to underestimate its scale at the outset, but all responded by increasing both the scope and the sophistication of their strategies. Then once changes had begun to occur, they had also to manage not only planned but also unplanned change. Additionally, as noted above, project managers lacked the authority to implement important developments according to timetable and so often had to reschedule. In general, sites retained the core of their plans but adjusted both the emphases they placed on different elements of RM and details of their implementation timetables.

CONCLUSION

The general picture that emerges of the planning and management of RM implementation is that both scope and quality increased over the period of the study. Progressively clearer plans and timetables led to a better understanding of the nature of RM and its links to wider organisational processes on the part of those involved. This suggests that while the sites might have benefitted from stronger project management, RM represents an advance on many projects conducted in the NHS in the early 1980s (National Audit Office, 1990). This said, it became evident that the planning process could not be extended to all aspects of RM, and the oft-reported lack of authority of project managers militated somewhat against their ability to keep to their timetables for implementation. To a significant extent, then, RM depended for its successful implementation on the trust and goodwill of all those involved.

Chapter 3

THE IMPLEMENTATION OF RM

INTRODUCTION

One of the most striking features of the pilot sites is the magnitude of the effort that has been directed to implementing RM. Staff from many parts of the hospital, supported by people with particular expertise from outside, have made very considerable personal investments in RM. Observation of the implementation process and interviews with many of the staff involved in it have revealed the scale and complexity of the task they undertook. In this chapter we discuss the implementation of RM. The progress made by the sites is considered under three broad headings: information and information systems; organisation and structure; and organisation development. In some instances, notably in relation to information systems, sites adopted quite distinctive approaches, and some of the differences both in overall emphasis and in the finer detail of implementation are highlighted where appropriate. Elsewhere though, the focus, as in other chapters, is on the RM Initiative as a whole, and examples are drawn from sites in order to illustrate general points.

INFORMATION AND INFORMATION SYSTEMS

One of the principal tasks of the RM project teams was to manage the design and implementation of new information systems. The elements of these systems - computerised databases, care profiles, clinical codes, budgets, training programmes - should not be confused with the RM process: they are part of the infrastructure deemed necessary to support the process. The sites have made major investments in them, and here we review the progress made with their design and implementation.

All of the sites had a variety of manual and computerised information systems in place at the start of the Initiative. They all had systems for collecting data for national requirements, although with the implementation of Körner from 1987-88 these were being reviewed. As noted in Chapter 1, four of the sites had been involved in earlier Management or Clinical Budgeting initiatives. But the sites varied in the extent to which they had computerised operational systems in place, with the Royal Hampshire and Arrowe Park having few and others having several which would be used throughout the experiment. None, however, had a central, integrated database with detailed individual patient data of the type envisaged in HN(86)34.

Computer systems for RM

The computer system most closely associated with RM is the RM database, also referred to as the case mix database. The Health Notice announcing RM stated that sites would implement databases, and indicated that the Department of Health attached importance to their development. They would be central, integrated systems which would support the work of managers and clinicians, both in the planning and review of work. Box 3.1 outlines the principal assumptions that underlay the sites' choice of systems and the data that they would contain. While all six sites developed RM databases, with the bulk of data derived from operational systems in wards and departments, they varied in the design adopted and in progress with implementation.

The two sites which undertook the initial design work were Freeman and Huddersfield. Freeman adopted a pragmatic approach, and implemented a database management system designed initially to provide data to staff at unit and sub-unit levels about in-patient activity - that is, the data most readily available in existing computer systems which could be transferred to the new central database. Reports generated on a routine basis comprised summary data on patient activity.

At Huddersfield, the system was also initially implemented for in-patient data, but was designed expressly with the clinical needs of individual consultants in mind. It contained the same basic patient activity data as the Freeman system, and additional details of resource use (tests ordered, test results, etc). Reporting screens were designed in collaboration with individual consultants, and were tailored to their requirements. Arrowe Park implemented a RM database which was similar to the Huddersfield design, but which was fed data from a ward ordering/results reporting system - that is, a Hospital Information System, or HIS.

Three of the other sites adopted systems similar to those developed by the two pioneers. Guy's and the Royal Hampshire followed a path similar to the Freeman's: both sites made considerable progress, but neither system was complete with respect to in-patient data by the end of the study. Arrowe Park selected a system similar to that at Huddersfield, which was just being implemented at the end of the study. The site which opted for a slightly different design solution was Pilgrim, where the strategy was to implement a system which was integrated closely with operational systems. Again, this was still under development at the end of the study, but was largely implemented with respect to in-patient activity data.

With the exception of Huddersfield, the sites intended in the future to implement separate, local databases for clinical review: this arises from local perceptions of the

Box 3.1   The RM database

Assumptions about the technology

1. Database software, on a mini or mainframe computer, is appropriate.

2. The database can be linked to operational systems: the data 'islands' can be joined.

3. A centralised database will be used by non-computer professionals to enter, manipulate and retrieve data.

4. The running costs are affordable.

Assumptions about the data

1. Most operational data required is already available.

2. Operational data is sufficiently accurate and complete to be passed to the RM database: the validation 'overhead' will be low.

3. Detailed individual patient activity data is required which can be aggregated and costed for use by managers and service providers.

4. It will be used, by different people for different purposes.

distinction between RM as against audit and other clinical review processes, and a desire to ensure local ownership of audit systems. In each case, however, it seems likely that data will be passed in both directions between the systems.

Turning from the databases to the operational systems which supply them, the sites again differed (Boxes 3.2 and 3.3). The principal of the overall design of the information systems is that selected data from operational systems is fed on a regular basis into the RM databases. Broadly, the sites followed one of two strategies in linking operational systems to the RM databases. At the Royal Hampshire wards and departments were linked by a HIS. Data from the system was passed daily across a single link to the RM database. The principal purpose of the system is to automate a wide range of activities in wards and departments.

The core of the system, for admissions, transfers and discharges, was designed with the aid of management consultants, but the largest and most technically difficult phase of implementation, covering the ordering and reporting functions, was implemented principally by NHS staff. The whole system was designed (that is to say, Anglicised from an American original) and implemented rapidly, and perhaps inevitably there were teething problems, some of them severe. At the end of the study the system was in place but still being refined.

At the other sites, individual departmental systems (typically already present before the RM database was designed) were linked individually to the RM databases, the intention being to build upon proven operational systems in preference to scrapping them and starting again.

At Guy's, a hospital network had also been installed which had results reporting facilities, allowing ward staff to access departmental systems (e.g. pathology and radiology) from ward-based terminals. The other sites had plans to go down a similar route: Pilgrim, for example, had the facilities in place for a network, but it had not so far been activated.

Whichever of these approaches the sites adopted, they found that implementing systems to the point where data from the operational systems could be passed regularly to the RM databases, could be validated therein, and reports then generated, took much longer than they had initially imagined. This reflects to a large extent the experimental nature of the implementation, where a variety of technical problems were encountered and the sites had to learn as they went. Sites also reported that they lacked sufficient NHS staff to cope with such a large-scale implementation. Taken together, this meant that often the flow of data to units and sub-units got worse before it got better, as old systems were abandoned and new systems delayed in implementation.

Box 3.2 Data from operational systems available in RM databases, summer 1990

	In-patient data	Pathology	Radiology	Pharmacy	Nursing (workload/dependency)	Theatres
Royal Hampshire	✓	X	X	X	X	X
Freeman	✓	✓	✓	X	X	✓
Guy's	✓	✓	✓	X	✓	✓
Huddersfield	✓	✓	✓	✓	X	✓
Pilgrim	✓	✓	✓	X	✓	✓

Wirral: RM database implemented in autumn 1990, with in-patient data (from a HIS) and pathology the first linked operational systems.

Box 3.3   Layout of principal computer systems

1. Freeman, Guy's, Huddersfield and Pilgrim

2. Arrowe Park and Royal Hampshire

Activity data

Box 3.4 shows that the quality of data in the RM databases was good, but that this was achieved in most sites only towards the end of the study. At each site, reasonable levels of accuracy and completeness were achieved from an initially low base. There are two ways in which this was tackled. First, the databases incorporated validation procedures, for checking data passed from operational systems, which were successively refined. Second, major efforts were made to ensure that staff recorded data correctly in the first place. This involved staff throughout the hospital: clerks in entering correct patient details, junior doctors in filling out test orders completely, and so on.

Across the sites, the use of data from the RM databases was variable. It was used at unit level to support the annual planning cycle, and for other purposes such as NHS Trust applications, and unit managers reported that it provided them with a valuable detailed overview of hospital activity such as they had never previously been able to obtain. At sub-unit level, though, there was a wide range of experiences from those where data was available and reviewed, through those where data was available but not being used, to those where it was desired but could not be obtained from the RM database (see Box 3.5). Some sub-unit heads at some sites received both routine and *ad hoc* reports, but these tended to be limited in scope. Similarly, data was available to individual service providers at some sites and not others. At some places it was actively used by some consultants, but others reported that they had yet to see a report relating to their own work.

Coding and patient classification

Clinical coding was tackled in different ways by the sites. In terms of organisation, coding was devolved to sub-unit level at all sites other than Guy's, where it remained centralised. The task of coding was thus redesigned, and much more than hitherto in the NHS, was a cooperative venture between coders and consultants and junior doctors. Within sub-units, however, there was variation both between and within sites. At Pilgrim Hospital, consultants met every week with coders to review codes, in Huddersfield, medical secretaries coded in-patient episodes, with varying consultant involvement; and so on. The degree to which consultants were involved varied considerably, with some seeing coding as crucial to their ability to review their work, and others totally uninterested.

The backbone of diagnostic coding in the UK is ICD-9, which is used for returns to the Department of Health. Locally, three sites currently use ICD-9-CM, and three use Read; both map to ICD-9 for central returns. Huddersfield was the first

Box 3.4   Accuracy and completeness of data in RM databases

Freeman

Comparison of the manual daily ward returns with the RM database showed that the percentages of in-patients recorded in the latter exceeded 98 per cent from the summer of 1989 onwards. For the pathology systems, the error rates (including all sources of errors) decreased sharply from mid-1989, e.g. for haematology the rate fell from 55.4 per cent in July 1989 to 15.9 per cent in July 1990.

Guy's

Not available.

Huddersfield

The hospital achieved 100 per cent agreement between all feeder systems and the RM database, through following up all discrepancies within one-two days of their occurrence.

Pilgrim

The agreement between operational systems and the RM database was low until mid-1990, at only 30-40 per cent for pathology, and 80 per cent for theatres for example. The principal reason for this was that previously the RM database had no facility for correcting errors. A software upgrade allowing error correction improved the situation from July 1990, and in the autumn the figure for theatres was 99 per cent, though the figure for pathology remained in the 30-40 per cent range. The agreement between PAS and the RM database, once very low, jumped to around 98 per cent by the end of the study.

Royal Hampshire

The completeness of data from the HIS steadily improved during the second half of 1989, but by early 1990 some 15 per cent of data was still being lost each month. 2-3 per cent was not recorded, 5-7 per cent was lost between the ward order/results reporting system and the RM database, and the remainder between software programs within the RM database. Latterly, the total data lost was reduced to around 1 per cent, principally through refinement of the system links and of the RM database software.

Box 3.5   RM databases at sub-unit level

The use of data from RM databases at sub-unit level was highly variable. There were a number of factors involved, which differed both within and between sites: they were successfully addressed in some places but not in others.

1. Provision or (perceived) availability of data to sub-unit staff.

2. Data present in the RM database but simple reports based on that data could not be produced or produced only with difficulty.

3. Perceived relevance of data, particularly for clinical review.

4. Perceptions of sub-unit staff of the accuracy of data with regard to review of clinical work.

5. Interest of staff in reports received: they were passive recipients of reports from unit level, and appeared to lack incentives to use them.

to adopt Read, and was later joined by Arrowe Park and Pilgrim. The exposure of a body of consultants to ICD-9 and ICD-9-CM provided invaluable information on their use within hospitals, though their experiences were mixed, with some specialties apparently well catered for and others much less so.

The Read system was developed by James Read, a GP based in Loughborough. It was recommended for use by GPs by the Royal College of General Practitioners (RCGP, 1989), and has subsequently been purchased by the Department of Health. During the period of the study, it was still under development, and had yet to be formally validated against ICD-9. Huddersfield was the first hospital in Britain to introduce it across all specialities. Read seemed to be generally popular with the Huddersfield consultants, several of whom had devoted considerable time to its implementation. Some had developed their own, local 'bibles' of codes specific to them within the Read framework. On the basis of experience at the sites to date, however, neither system could be said to be superior to the other.

Turning to patient classification, HN(86)34 stated that RM would involve, 'experimenting with the use of diagnostic related groups (DRGs) and other approaches to case mix planning'. Department of Health representatives have co-ordinated developments in this area. During the first two years of the Initiative, consultants at the sites examined DRGs relevant to their specialties, principally to determine to what extent they were clinically meaningful and predictive of resource use in the context of health care delivery in the NHS (with length of stay a proxy for resource use). Broadly, they found that some DRGs were both meaningful to clinicians and closely described resource use, others might with some refinement fulfil these criteria, and others were simply not useful in the context of the NHS. By and large, neither DRGs nor any other patient classification system were used routinely at the sites (though Freeman is to some extent an exception here).

It should also be noted here that work was undertaken on the development of outcome measures at some sites. However, involvement was patchy, and most work in this area remained experimental.

Care profiles

The Case Mix Management System Core Specification (Department of Health, 1989c) included a requirement that RM databases have facilities for care profiles. The sites varied both in their adherence to this requirement and in their interpretation of what care profiles comprised.

Their development was most advanced in Huddersfield, where from the outset they were built into the RM database for use by clinicians. They consisted of the expected pattern of care for a given type of patient, typically derived from consultants' own historical treatment patterns, or from a conscious exercise in designing the most appropriate pattern of care, drawing on available literature, judgements of colleagues, and so on. These profiles could then be compared with actual patterns of treatment, as part of consultants' review of their work. Deviations of actual from expected patterns could in principle be used either to change the treatment of future cases, or to review the validity of the profile.

At other sites progress was more limited. A research project was in progress at Freeman Hospital for most of the period of this study, in collaboration with Clinical Accountability, Service Planning and Evaluation (CASPE) of the King's Fund College, where consultants in a number of specialties were developing protocols for a range of conditions. Detailed data were collected on treatment patterns, patient satisfaction and post-discharge health status, and were being used to develop formal protocols. The Royal Hampshire was in the early stages of work intended to design multi-disciplinary care profiles, where the profiles contained expected treatment patterns and resource use, for nurses and professions allied to medicine as well as consultants. It was intended that this would facilitate coordinated care on the wards and multi-disciplinary review of care, and contribute to medical audit.

Nurses at all six sites developed care profiles, typically independently of consultants. Generally, they were designed for use in planning and review of care over either a given 24-hour period or an in-patient stay. Again, they were at different stages of development by the end of the study, some sites having them for all or most wards, others only for some. One noteworthy point here is that some sites (e.g. Guy's) developed theirs centrally, while others (e.g. in the medicine sub-unit at the Royal Hampshire) developed them more locally.

Nursing systems

Each of the six sites invested in computer systems for use by nursing staff, the development of which was typically undertaken as a sub-project of the main RM project. It has been noted on many occasions that the development of such systems can be particularly problematic (DHSS, 1985; Bagust, 1989; Department of Health, 1990b), and there is no generally accepted blueprint for their design, although there is now guidance available on system selection and implementation (Department of Health, 1990b; NHSTA, 1990).

The most striking single point about the nursing projects was the focus on computerisation. There were a number of reasons given by the sites for computerising: nursing activity could be better matched to workload; it would make care delivery more systematic; automating care planning would save nursing time; the RM databases required data from ward-based feeder systems; it would facilitate costing of nursing activity; and so on. This was reflected in the systems selected and implemented.

In practice, each site began by adopting an existing method for estimating dependency and workload, and either computerised it themselves or purchased systems which incorporated the desired method. To a large extent, this seemed to have happened principally because the systems were available, and other systems would take more development work. Latterly, some sites implemented new rostering systems. All sites implemented at least one system, but progress was slower than initially anticipated, at least by the members of nursing project teams.

Not the least reason for this was that implementation was subject to a range of technical problems, which in many ways were typical of problems experienced with systems more generally. At the Freeman, for example, problems stemmed from the main computer system being based at another hospital. When the links between the two hospitals were planned, their capacity allowed for the running of systems on only ten wards. An upgrade was planned in 1989, but had not yet been installed by the end of the study, with the result that no more wards could yet be computerised. Moreover, there remained problems with the reliability of the system, and all wards still used manual systems in parallel.

The Royal Hampshire's HIS (later also adopted by Arrowe Park) was designed to automate a wide range of nursing (as well as clinical and clerical) activities, and included a range of facilities from tools for patient assessment and planning of care to supplies ordering. Clearly, it had a profound effect at ward level. Nurses accepted the principle that the system could help them to deliver better care, but felt that in practice it was very demanding of nursing time, with no provision of the necessary clerical support.

Other sites also experienced technical problems, and in this regard it is noteworthy that only two sites had their main systems linked to the RM database during 1990 (see Box 3.2). Given that computerisation was a major focus of the efforts of nursing project teams, the sites produced little evidence that their assumptions about computerisation were justified, and ward sisters were in general cynical about the systems. At Huddersfield, for example, they reported that computerising care planning took more rather than less time, than with their former manual system. Claims that it would provide more accurate data were denied, with reports from some sites that during busy periods recording of activity went by the wayside.

It is not clear whether these problems at ward level were due to the properties of the systems or the way in which they were implemented. It does, though, emphasise that while nurses chose the systems, this was often not done in collaboration with ward-based staff. Rather, assumptions were made by senior nurses about the nature of activities at ward level, and what information nurses there would find useful. The reaction of ward sisters at several sites was that they felt systems had been imposed on them, and that they lacked relevance to their work. Others, however, did feel involved in system selection, but still reported frustration with technical problems.

> Poor quality of documentation, i.e. the ward staff have gone from working hard to produce excellent handwritten care plans to printing out trash.
>
> Ward Sister

More generally, sites did not first work out their information needs, and so focused on a relatively narrow range of issues. Inevitably, this is reflected in patchy developments at all sites; there have been some isolated successes, with a few reports of the quality of data improving. But in general there is little to show for a great deal of effort in this area.

Development of budgets

One of the original purposes of the RM Initiative was to develop 'patient case mix planning and costing', by 'strengthening the existing specialty costing and planning systems ... linking the financial and activity systems together into a key-item planning and reporting system' (DHSS, 1986a). This reflected the Department of Health's desire to build upon the progress made by some of the Management Budgeting sites, and confirms the commitment to specialty costing recommended by the Körner Steering Committee (DHSS, 1982-84). The sites were thus charged with establishing how activities and costs could be linked.

With regard to the budgets used within the hospitals, these typically comprised management budgets. These were devolved to sub-units, consistent with devolution of responsibility for their management. Sub-unit staff were in frequent contact with their finance departments about the accuracy of statements (see Box 6.2): as a result of these discussions the accuracy of statements increased over the course of the Initiative, though the extent to which sub-unit staff trusted them varied. Nevertheless, these statements allowed sub-unit staff to investigate the relationships, in the aggregate, between activities and costs. At two sites - Freeman and Royal Hampshire - budgets were further devolved to ward level. Elsewhere, ward level budgets were produced within finance departments but since budgetary responsibility had not been devolved, they were not used in management processes at this level.

It is at ward level, though, that some of the key issues for RM were brought into sharp relief, as the quote below illustrates.

> We will be told the medical unit is very much overspent, and that it is you, the ward sisters with your budget that are causing a lot of this overspending, and what are you going to do about it? How are you going to cut back? So we do take the responsibility. On the other hand, we have to stand for the patient and say, 'look, we are giving the best possible care that we can, but the staff are really working flat out all the time.'
>
> Sister Anne Hammersley
> Royal Hampshire, on
> *Business Matters*, BBC2,
> 27 September 1990

During 1989 and 1990, sites began to calculate costs with the aim of being able to cost activity to individual patient level. These calculations were either retained in manual form, or entered into the RM database but held separately from activity data. Towards the end of the study, some sites began to investigate cost and volume variances, at individual patient level.

However, linking activities and costs at this level depends on having accurate activity data available. As discussed above, sites devoted considerable efforts to ensuring that activity data was accurate, and it was only during 1990 that it became accurate enough to cost for the purpose of constructing budgets.

Some sites cited other reasons for not having made more rapid progress with costing. During 1989 and early 1990 some sites reported that they were unsure what approaches to costing were best suited to developing block and other contracts, and so consciously did not commit themselves to expenditure on the development of new systems or new approaches to costing. Regions indicated that hospitals would be required to negotiate only block contracts during 1991-92, using average specialty costs. This meant that the more detailed data required for cost and volume and individual patient contracts was not required, and detailed understanding of cost and volume variances would not be necessary until at least early 1992. Some sites were thus delaying work in this area.

In general, then, the major thrust of developments in information systems in RM was concerned with the design of systems for collecting activity data, and ensuring that the data was accurate, rather than on the costing of that activity. However, sites refined existing management budgeting systems over the course of the study, and these were increasingly used at sub-unit level.

Training

All of the sites organised courses for staff, which typically focused on the use of computer hardware and software and other formal skills. Initially, existing hospital staff who were to use a system had to be trained, and then provision made for new staff. The organisation and quantity of training provided varied greatly between sites. A highly structured approach was taken at the Royal Hampshire and Arrowe Park, staff at those sites feeling that the scale of their computer system implementations made it essential. Indeed, training was regarded locally as being a central plank of RM implementation. At other sites training had a less central role; it was less formalised, consisting typically of a mixture of programmed and *ad hoc* courses and meetings.

Evidence on training from three groups - ward sisters, coders and business managers - suggests that what was provided was in general appropriate, but there was not nearly enough of it. The sites were acutely aware of this, but were not able to provide it to the levels they would themselves have desired: only some staff at Arrowe Park reported that their training was appropriate to the requirements of RM.

In comments in their questionnaires, ward sisters at all sites reported that there was training in the use of computers, but that it was inadequate. They felt that the initial training they were given was useful, but that they did not receive enough support over the following weeks and months. This could not have been due to a lack of effort on the part of those responsible for training, who at times felt under enormous strain from the demands of staff.

Coders undoubtedly moved from obscurity into full view at several of the sites. This focused attention on the nature of the coding process and the training necessary for coders. The sites were deeply divided on this issue. Sites such as Pilgrim asserted that coding was a distinct skill, and coding staff were a valuable resource who justified training and support. Huddersfield took a similar view, but believed that the level of skill required meant that only medical secretaries (at least from among administrative and clerical staff) had the knowledge to code cases accurately. The Freeman and Guy's, on the other hand, whilst recognising that coding was a skilled activity, also felt that it could be automated, and had introduced PC-based software which could be used to assign ICD-9-CM codes on the basis of primary and secondary diagnoses. Whether coding is or is not automated, coding staff need training. But the whole approach to this training differs, one strategy is aimed at investing solely in people, the other much less so. This example illustrates the fact that even after four years the sites differed significantly in their views on some elements of RM.

Business managers require a considerable range of formal and informal skills. Generally, the training and support provided has been highly variable and relatively limited. It appears that business managers were expected to learn RM 'on the job': indeed, this was viewed by unit managers as both desirable and unavoidable. But in most cases the business managers, themselves, reported that they felt undereducated in formal skills relevant to their jobs, notably in the ability to manipulate data in the RM databases and generate reports from them.

A feature common to the sites, then, seems to be a lack of resources available for training and support, and a relatively narrow focus on computers at the expense of broader issues.

ORGANISATION AND STRUCTURE

Sub-unit organisation, in the form of both the medical specialty groupings that determined clinical priorities and provided management with advice, and the functional groupings of wards for nursing management, predated RM. Indeed two of the three experimental sites that now have a comprehensive clinical directorate structure at sub-unit level had moved to this pattern of organisation before the RM Initiative commenced. So sub-unit organisational structure was not a creation of RM. It appears however, that it is a necessary component.

This association is hardly surprising. Service providers' willingness to become involved in management was laid down as a pre-condition for a site to be included in the experiment, and the creation of a sub-unit structure is an obvious manifestation of commitment. And as the RM experiment continued so it became apparent that some form of comprehensive sub-unit organisational structure, that brought together those engaged in caring for particular groups of patients, was necessary if service providers were to engage with the RM process. (Although in practice some service divisions are organised on the basis of services that support the care provided to all patients, such as pathology or radiology.) The organisation of service providers has moved towards the clinical directorate model. This divides the unit into a number of multi-disciplinary groupings according to the main work outputs, whereas the traditional model of unit organisation which it replaced was based upon single disciplinary hierarchies and representative mechanisms that reflected staff inputs. The difference is depicted in Box 3.6.

Box 3.6   Models of unit organisation

1. Traditional

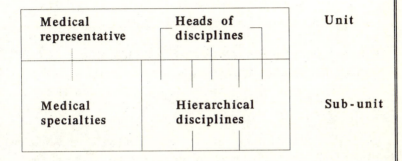

2. Directorate

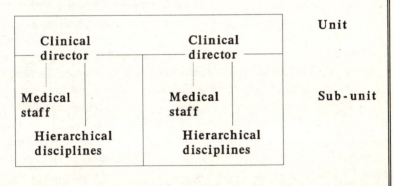

At the time of our Interim Report in mid-1989 Arrowe Park, Guy's and the Royal Hampshire hospitals were already strongly committed to the directorate model, which they claimed was an essential component of RM. The other three sites were less certain. They had not approached RM by a structural route and although they saw clinical directorates as one possibility, there were others and they were keen to let the structure evolve.

> If doctors and management in a hospital have good relationships (as we have) then there is no need to meddle with the system.
>
> Consultant

By the end of 1990 the process of evolution had, in fact, taken the Freeman, Huddersfield and Pilgrim hospitals significantly nearer to directorates, although they would not necessarily wish to use the title or adopt all the properties of a full-blown directorate. Our respondents saw directorates as offering attractions to both general managers and service providers. To the former they provided convenient groupings for the devolution of central authority, bringing managers in touch with the prime activities of patient care in a way that had hitherto been impossible, or only achievable with the expenditure of enormous energy and charisma. The presence of directorates as units of management also eased the whole process of creating and meeting service contracts that was required by the new legislation, providing a convenient entity for calculating costs. For the service providers, directorates provided a ready focus for RM in that they were made up of staff who held shared interests and required common information. In many cases the directorates mirrored specialty and ward groupings and thus respected historic boundaries. Bringing the service providers together provided a platform for developing more flexible services and gave their particular interests greater clout within the wider unit. Clearly they received added encouragement from the new legislation which required clinicians within specialties to collaborate in order to undertake medical audit. The Central Consultants and Specialists Committee gave clinical directorates cautious approval in their evaluation of the experimental sites (CCSC, 1989):

> it may prove a constructive way for consultants to play a proper role in the management of hospitals, thus ensuring the best use of resources for patient care.

But other respondents, particularly in the non-directorate sites, argued that RM operated to strengthen both the ability of individual service providers to manage their own activities and of unit managers to manage collective activities. It followed that a strong sub-unit management role would be unnecessary, although sub-units would be helpful for co-ordinating individual activities and aggregating advice for unit managers.

The properties of sub-unit structures

Box 3.7 lists some of the properties that might be expected in a service directorate. Box 3.8 that follows lists some of the differences between the sites in the way in which their own sub-units meet these properties. It must be stressed that our analysis is based upon our generalised perceptions of developments at the six sites over the period of the experiment and may not accord with individual perceptions, contractual obligations or local assumptions, all of which are likely to differ. If, on the face of it, the degree of conformity is impressive, divergences begin to appear when the terms are unpacked.

1. *The number and type of sub-unit divisions.* This is clearly partly a function of size. The larger the number of service providers and the larger the amount of resources involved, the more divisions will be needed. For if the divisions are too large the advantages of common interests will be lost and they will pose an impossible management task for a part-time director. Guy's, as a large teaching hospital, found it necessary to create a sub-directorate level of management which they termed Clinical Groups.

   A second consideration is the type of services that are provided. A ready distinction can be made between those services that determine clinical care and those, such as radiology and pathology that support the care determined by others. Small specialist services not large enough to form a directorate in their own right, are harder to place.

   Yet a third consideration is the history of how specialties and disciplines have been grouped in the past, and the presence or absence of individuals who appear committed and capable of taking on a managerial role.

2. *Allocation of a budget to the divisions.* If the divisions are to have a meaningful role in managing their own resources they require their own budget. Where sites have sub-unit divisions, they now all receive a budget allocation, although the proportion of unit funds that are allocated down varies between the sites, as does the process by which the size of the budget is determined.

Box 3.7   Properties of service directorates

1. Units divided into areas by service output.

2. Unit budget allocated to service areas.

3. Appointment of a practising service provider as head.

4. Head is answerable for services provided.

5. Head has authority to lead the work of staff providing services.

6. Head is held accountable for the application of the budget provided.

7. Head receives managerial support.

8. Head participates in corporate unit management.

Box 3.8 Properties of sub-units in the six sites - autumn 1990

	Arrowe Park	Freeman	Guy's	Huddersfield	Pilgrim	Royal Hampshire
1. Units divided into areas by service outputs	15 directorates	10 clinical specialties + sub-groups	15 directorates + clinical groups	3 clinical service groups	Not comprehensively, 4 pilot directorates	8 directorates
2. Unit budget allocated to service areas	✓	✓	✓ directorates and clinical groups	✓	✓ (in pilots)	✓
3. Appointment of a practising service provider as Head	Consultant	Consultant	Consultant	Consultant	Consultant (in pilots)	Consultant
4. Head is answerable for services provided	✓	✓	✓	✓	✓ (in pilots)	✓
5. Head has authority to lead the work of staff providing services	✓	✓	✓	✓	✓ (in pilots)	✓
6. Head is held accountable for the application of the budget provided	✓	✓	✓	✓	✓ (in pilots)	✓
7. Head receives managerial support	Business & Nursing Managers	Specialty Manager	Business & Nursing Managers	Resource Services Manager	Business & Nursing Managers (in pilots)	Buisness & Nursing Managers
8. Head participates in corporate unit management	Hospital Council	via UGM & Medical Executive	Hospital Management Board	Policy Advisory Board	via UGM & Medical representatives	Unit Management Board

3. *Appointment of a service provider as head of the division.* It has been a principle of the directorate model that the head must be actively engaged in delivering services to patients, thereby demonstrating that service providers can engage in management, and maintaining common interests and credibility with his, or her, fellow practitioners. Heads of division report that their work occupies at least one and as many as four half-day sessions over a week, and that it displays an ability to expand to fill all available time.

In general the heads have been limited to consultants; although Arrowe Park has had experience with two non-medical directors, all directors there will be consultants from April 1991.

The appointment of a head displays all the characteristics of religious preferment. The usual method appears to be the emergence of a candidate who is willing to take the job and who is acceptable to both the consultant members of the division and the UGM, with either of the two parties being able to initiate the process.

4. *The answerability of the head for the work of the division.* Without doubt heads of divisions are generally regarded as answerable for their divisions; providing points of contact and explanation. Whether this extends to their personally being held to account for activities that are performed by other members depends on the nature of their authority as leaders.

5. *The authority of the head to lead staff in the division.* Where there are heads of division, they are certainly expected to lead their divisions although the attributes of leadership are not precisely defined. The authority to lead can be seen as potentially occupying a range of relationships from direction at the full managerial extreme, through co-ordination and monitoring of activities, to advice at the non-managerial extreme. The situation regarding other clinicians in the division is, in general, that the head is 'the first among equals', expected to co-ordinate and monitor activities. With the non-clinical staff it was suggested at Freeman that the head of the clinical specialty had authority to direct their work. In two further sites, Arrowe Park and Royal Hampshire, a directive relationship was also felt to exist, although this was in respect of day to day operational work, professional matters remaining the responsibility of senior officers in the disciplines concerned. In the other sites non-clinical staff were seen as being directed by their own senior officers, although aspects of their work were co-ordinated and monitored by heads of divisions. In the absence of the authority to direct the work of members of divisions, heads can hardly be held accountable for their performance.

6. *The accountability of the head of division for the application of the allocated budget.*
In all cases where units are divided into service divisions and these are allocated
budgets, the head of the division is regarded as accountable for their budget. In
some cases budgetary accountability is sub-divided to lower levels or according to
particular functions. The senior nurse manager, or managers are likely to be
made accountable for the nursing budget and aspects of this may be delegated
further to ward sisters. But in many cases, especially where the divisional
structure is a recent initiative, heads appear as unsure as to what their budgetary
accountability actually means and what discretion they have to alter expenditure
between different items.

7. *The presence of managerial support.* Given that it is a principle that the head of
the division is a most-time practitioner and minor-time manager, respondents see
it as vital that he or she receives some full-time support. This is needed in two
areas. First, to direct the day to day work of the considerable number of non-
clinical staff. And second, to act as a staff officer, collecting and interpreting the
information through which the division is managed, monitoring the achievement
of objectives, taking a lead in planning the future activities of the division, and
acting as a point of negotiation with individual members of the division, with
other divisions and with unit managers. The former support is generally supplied
by a nursing manager or senior nursing officer, the latter by a business manager
or general services manager. There was considerable debate in the early stages
of RM whether this support required one role or two. Majority opinion now
favours the latter option so the roles are treated separately below:

   (a) the nurse manager is, as the title suggests, the head of the nursing hierarchy
   within the sub-unit and may also be made manager of other non-clinical and
   non-clerical staff within the division. As manager of these key resources the
   nurse manager carries some accountability to the head of division, although
   the latter may occupy a co-ordinating rather than a directive relationship. In
   any case professional accountability for the nursing aspect of the work is
   typically outside the sub-unit to a unit nursing role. As is well illustrated by
   the draft specification in Box 3.9; the nurse manager is also likely to be
   involved in other aspects of RM. Where the nurse manager and business
   manager roles are combined, as with specialty managers at Freeman, the
   occupant is preferably but not necessarily a nurse;

   (b) the business manager provides the necessary management expertise,
   particularly as assistant to the head of the division, but also to other
   members. The business manager runs the division's office, if there is such a

Box 3.9   An example of the role of a nurse manager in a sub-unit

The senior nurse manager

To provide professional and managerial leadership, primarily to own unit but also throughout the acute area when the need arises.

To advise the clinical director on the best use of nursing staff to provide an efficient and cost effective service, ensuring the highest possible standards of care are provided.

Accountability:

- Director of nursing services on all professional issues.

- Clinical director for all day to day issues on own unit.

Authority:

- Line manager for nursing staff.

- Appointing staff up to RN level as delegated by director of nursing services.

- Assuring professional and managerial development of all nursing staff.

- Functional authority over non-nursing staff when patient care issues are involved.

Key areas:

The nurse manager works closely with the business manager to ensure that the needs of the division are met with particular emphasis on:

- Ensuring the highest possible environmental and care standards.

- Management of non-medical and non-nursing staff including advice on cost effective cover for absence taking into account above.

- Giving help regarding patient statistics and other relevant information needed to efficiently manage the division.

- Maintaining and improving communication within the unit, ensuring the director has all the information and assistance required to effectively manage the unit.

facility, and directs the work of the clerical staff. The draft specification listed in Box 3.10 is only one of a number of versions of its kind but it does give an indication of what is involved in these roles. Business mangers can be thought of as a bridge between the sub-unit and the wider unit. However the role may be unit based, providing a service to sub-units and monitoring their activities on behalf of the unit, or, more commonly based in the sub-unit, and either fully accountable to the head or operationally accountable to the head and professionally accountable to a unit management role. The precise arrangements are likely to give rise to different views of the business managers prime loyalty. Business managers have proved particularly scarce on the ground during the development of RM, but their skills, if originally regarded with scepticism by some service providers, have come to be seen as crucial to the success of devolution. As the RM Initiative has proceeded, so the scope of their roles has enlarged, taking on, for example, marketing and financial advisory roles. This strengthens the capacity and freedom of divisions and can be balanced by a reduction in the work formerly carried out by unit based managers.

8. *Nature of participation of heads of divisions in unit management.* It appears to be a property of the clinical directorate structure that there is an executive board or council that brings all the directors together with the UGM and other senior unit managers, to consider the corporate policy and conduct of the unit. This is the case at Arrowe Park, Guy's and the Royal Hampshire. In the other sites where clinical directorates do not exist or are in the course of development, sub-unit participation in unit management is less clear-cut, exercised through advisory bodies that are separate from the unit management executive or through the traditional routes of medical representation and functional management. This is more the pattern that was found at Freeman, Huddersfield and Pilgrim.

It is possible to discern two different constitutional viewpoints with regard to devolution of authority to sub-units by unit management. The first could be termed the confederate model. If devolution is to be a reality, the interests of those bodies to whom authority is devolved have to be strongly expressed in unit management. The function of the latter is to aggregate, arbitrate and advance the interests of the service providers. Those who favour this position will press for strong unit management boards or councils, with all the heads of divisions as delegate members.

The second viewpoint could be termed the Federal model. Those functions that can be suitably devolved are left to the divisions, other functions cannot be devolved and remain the prerogative of unit management. The views of the divisions may be required to aid unit management but they can be obtained in

Box 3.10 An example of the role of a business manager (general services manager) in a sub-unit

1. *Accountability and relationships*

   Accountable to: director of clinical services

- Relates within the division to: senior nurse manager, consultant and other medical staff, heads of linked departments, ward sisters.

- Relates beyond the division to: other GSMs, senior officers - particularly finance manager and assistant UGM.

2. *Role and functions*

   The GSM's major role is to support the director of clinical services in his management responsibilities.

   In fulfilling this role the GSM's major functions will be to:

- Manage information services within the division. Specific tasks include:

   (a) ensuring that the collection, collation, analysis and presentation of information (activity, financial and manpower) is carried out in the division to standards that are commensurate with those set for the acute unit as a whole;

   (b) co-ordinating the implementation of information systems within the division, and managing the necessary trouble-shooting.

- Organise effective communication processes within the division. Specific tasks include facilitating the director's requirements for management meetings concerning the creation, implementation and monitoring of divisional plans, and identifying cross-divisional issues which may arise.

- Manage the non-medical and non-nursing staff accountable within the divisional office. Specific tasks include managing annual/sick leave cover economically within existing staff levels whenever possible.

- Organise the distribution and allocation of work within the divisional office. Specific tasks include creating and nurturing the correct level of clerical and secretarial support for the division as a whole.

- Agree annually with the director a programme of tasks and objectives personal to the GSM for the financial year.

a number of ways: by general managers; presented by elected representatives; by advisory mechanisms or, by head of divisions attending management board or councils. Unit decisions do not depend upon agreement by the divisions.

The former, Confederate model can be seen where sub-unit structures were motivated by the desire for the service providers to dominate management. The latter, Federal model can be seen where sub-unit structures were motivated by the desire of unit managers to get the service providers contributing to management. In practice the contribution of heads of divisions within the same site appears to oscillate between the two models according to the issues at stake.

Problems in involving service providers in management

The movement towards sub-unit organisation has not been without criticism, generally associated with the problem of grafting managerial authority and accountability on to clinicians, whose working practices are built around clinical freedom. The issues were analysed for the NHS Management Executive by the Institute of Health Service Management (Disken *et al.*, 1990). The then Director of the Institute was subsequently quoted as claiming that full-blown clinical directorates were 'a myth' in terms of directors exercising full responsibility for managing nursing and other non-clinical staff (*Health Service Journal*, 14 June 1990). It is our experience that the responsibilities of sub-units frequently appear clearer from outside, from the district or unit perspective, than from within. Staff working within sub-units are, understandably more aware of the limitations and of the presence of unresolved issues of authority and accountability. In the short-term these tend to be ignored, the problems they cause resolved on an *ad hoc* basis, because staff have an interest in making the new arrangements work. It was prophesied by individuals at the six sites that the imminent introduction of targets and business plans as part of the contractual process would be likely to fracture relationships and test the reality of accountability and authority (*Health Service Journal*, 14 June 1990) although others were less pessimistic. Boxes 3.11 and 3.12 draw upon these criticisms, as well as upon our own observations, to highlight some of the differences in the way in which the authority and accountability of heads of division are perceived.

Respondents saw a potential danger that if sub-units built up too strong an identify they might become parochial and/or baronial, not readily looking beyond their own interests. This was clearly a danger in the operation of unit-wide mechanisms such as management or advisory boards, but in the opinion of most respondents with a unit perspective the danger had not, often to their surprise, yet transpired. Heads of division had to consider the interests of their own practice as well as acting as delegates to promote the interests of their division, but they were

Box 3.11 The authority of the head of division

1. Full management

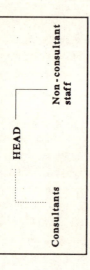

Head can direct the work of all the staff in the division. (Unlikely given consultants' clinical freedom.)

2. Part management

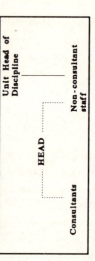

Head is accepted as co-ordinator rather than director of the work of consultants and can direct non-clinical staff. (The latter is difficult on a part-time and non-specialist basis.)

3. Shared management

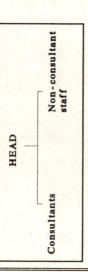

Head co-ordinates the work of the consultants. Direction of non-clinical staff is shared by the head (operational performance) and unit head of discipline (professional matters).

4. Non-management

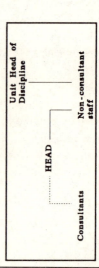

Head is essentially a co-ordinator rather than a manager of the work of division. Non-clinical staff are directed by senior officers in their own discipline, or float.

Box 3.12   The accountability of the head of division

1. To UGM

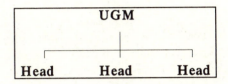

Heads of division are accountable to UGM's for their work in leading a division. The Unit Board is advisory to the UGM. (If heads are consultants, retaining their own practice, clinical freedom is likely to restrict the UGM's managerial relationship to divisional matters, or as proposed by the IHSM the relationship may be contractual.)

2. To Management Board

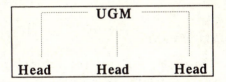

Heads of division are accountable to the board as a whole for their work in leading a division. As Chief Executive of the board the UGM can co-ordinate and monitor, but not fully direct, the work of heads.

also seen to be aware of wider constraints and interests. General managers were heartened that boards made up of heads of sub-units could reach agreement on priorities, as for new staff or locating expenditure cuts, that were not necessarily in the immediate interest of all concerned.

Other implications

The emergence of the sub-unit level of organisation is the most obvious structural change associated with RM, so it has received emphasis. The involvement of individual service providers in management activities is as, if not more, important but this is treated later. What does require mention here is that the development of sub-units must also effect the unit structures. It has already been mentioned that if unit functions are devolved, then it follows that unit personnel can also be re-located in the sub-units. We have observed that units are having to give more emphasis to providing supporting services and to co-ordinating and monitoring work; pulling together proposals from the divisions and integrating them in a unit plan; monitoring how far plans are implemented; monitoring expenditure; helping with the new technologies. These emphases have required changes in the way in which unit work is organised and in the content of unit roles. Unit managers have stressed the importance of being available to physically work with sub-unit managers to iron-out problems and boost motivation, at the expense of other traditional central management tasks.

ORGANISATION DEVELOPMENT

HN(86)34 emphasised that the pilot sites would spend time clarifying arrangements for involving doctors and nurses in management. Indeed, the sites were selected on the basis that doctors and nurses were already involved in management processes, and this would be built upon through 'management development and training programmes' (DHSS, 1986a). In practice, the nature and depth of involvement of doctors and nurses at the start of the experiment varied both within and between sites. At Guy's and the Royal Hampshire, sub-unit managers were clearly involved, but in general other clinicians and nurses were not. Elsewhere, there was less formal involvement, with attitudes of most service providers towards RM ranging from enthusiastic to agnostic, with only a few antagonists voicing their opinions.

The first stage of organisation development associated with RM was concerned with creating the conditions within hospitals to allow change to take place. At the start, the impetus for RM was provided by 'local champions', people with power within sites and a vision of how RM could transform the organisation. These were, variously, district chairmen, district and unit general managers and clinicians. These champions were able to enlist the support of others within the hospital, who did not necessarily share an identical vision but did share a perception that 'things' could in some way be improved. These groups, which were typically informal, were instrumental in creating the intellectual and cultural climate for change.

The nature of the arguments that were used at this stage to convince people of the merits of RM varied between sites, depending on local circumstances and the personalities involved. For example, in some cases it was suggested to clinicians that formal involvement in management would enable them to influence resource allocation more directly, or that information systems could be provided that would help them to review their own work or facilitate research. Managers were lobbied with arguments about the logic of clinical involvement, or with the promise of being better able to control the use of resources.

The major change associated with these discussions was the adoption of new organisation structures, as described in the previous section. During the course of the study, most sites were either developing their new structures or making the change, which offered an opportunity to observe developments at first hand. Two points relating to this major change stand out. First, the long term effects of changing organisation structures could not be foreseen. Thus while a theoretical case for new structures could be argued, to a significant extent the changes involved an act of faith for those involved. Second, the new structures implied a new distribution of power. It is instructive here to note that the main discussions were between unit managers and clinicians, with nurses tending to be marginalised. Senior staff at Huddersfield said that, given the opportunity again, they would implement their nursing systems earlier and integrate nursing development more closely with other elements of RM.

Conversely, it is striking that not everyone was initially affected by the changes. Clinical directors and nurse and business managers had to make the new structures work, and some administrative and clerical staff experienced substantial role changes, but other staff - notably clinicians and ward sisters - were largely unaffected. Many staff were thus able to avoid thinking about RM; and those directly involved initially committed themselves to general principles rather than to the detail of RM.

As the Initiative progressed, the sites came to appreciate the extent to which organisation development had to be linked to computer implementation strategies. At all of them most of the computer development work was carried out 'behind the scenes', by project teams and other computing and information staff. But sites differed in the extent to which staff in the body of the organisation were consulted. Broadly, there were two strategies. Huddersfield consciously emphasised the potential value of their RM database to individual clinicians in reviewing their work. Each clinician had the opportunity of having reporting screens designed to reflect his or her own needs. This was part of a broader strategy to involve clinicians in management processes. Other sites tended to consult less widely at the outset, though all had groups of clinicians advising on system design; here, routine reports or access to the database were offered once a set of standard reporting screens had been developed.

It became increasingly apparent that the ways in which organisation development could be managed were constrained both by the new organisation structures and by the need to timetable the implementation of information systems. RM involved change not only for clinicians and nurses, but also for unit and sub-unit managers and for other staff such as coders. The sites responded by rethinking their approaches, and increasing the numbers of staff who would be actively encouraged to participate in RM. This development was most marked at sub-unit level, and here we consider changes at two sites to illustrate key developments.

At the Freeman, new sub-unit structures were adopted in 1989, and some of the first sub-unit business meetings, which were held monthly, were observed. At the outset the participants (consultants, senior registrars and specialty managers) were unsure of their roles, and tended to discuss relatively minor issues. Very quickly, within two or three months, they began to discuss more substantive issues, such as the content of their sub-unit business plans, and were altogether more purposeful. There was little overt intervention over this period, and what appears to have happened is that sub-unit staff were working out their own ways of doing things. The way in which this occurred was in large part unplanned: they were learning management by doing it.

It was also apparent that RM evolved at different rates in different parts of the hospital. Thus some specialties adopted new ways of working more rapidly than others. Once the new structures had been adopted, to some extent sub-units could evolve independently.

Once change had begun to occur, the task was to sustain it. This depended on achieving a stable power structure. What happened next is exemplified by the Royal Hampshire, where directorates were already established at the start of the Initiative. Here, there were moves to formalise the development process, with the appointment of project managers and project teams, part of whose brief was organisation development; and change agents, who acted as facilitators with different groups of staff, and had a more general role as people who were available to talk over organisational issues. Local champions remained key figures, but were increasingly supported by these other staff.

At the Royal Hampshire (as at other sites), clinical directors, nurse managers and business managers all changed in their approaches to their own roles, and their relationships with one another. The clinical directors were heavily involved in unit and sub-unit processes, and over time their commitment strengthened to the point where they shared the championing of RM. They underwent very little formal training, and again learned on the job. Nurse managers, in contrast, tended to focus more narrowly on nursing-related issues. One reason for this was the scale of the changes affecting ward nurses, most obviously in the implementation of the HIS. A significant part of the job of nurse managers was thus directed to supporting ward-based nurses. The result, in general, was that nurse managers and nursing staff developed from within, but their external relationships with other staff groups changed relatively little. By and large nurses looked after their own organisation developments, though with additional support from a change agent.

Business managers were first appointed at the Royal Hampshire in 1987, and so the post was still a relatively new one. They quickly worked out both what they could do and in what directions their jobs might develop. But their jobs were defined in part in relation to the clinical director and nurse manager. Inevitably, perhaps, there were tensions. As their roles came to be understood, so the expectations of both unit management and consultants grew. The short history of the business manager has to a significant extent been the story of attempts to resolve these conflicts. The problems were recognised, as witnessed by the arrangement of away-days for business managers where their roles were discussed, but not satisfactorily resolved.

THE NATURE OF RM IMPLEMENTATION

The variety of approaches to implementation used at the sites, and their problems and achievements, allow for some general comments about the nature of the change processes associated with RM. By the end of the study period, the sites had undergone substantial organisational change, and key individuals had experienced substantial cultural change, which in some respects marked a radical departure from previous ways of working. While the nature of some of these changes must be regarded as part of the research and development work of the sites, and thus inherently experimental, it did seem that some elements of organisation development in RM would have occurred whatever the initial level of understanding of RM. This was the case particularly for the commitment of staff to RM, which visibly increased during the study; and also in the increased trust between members of different professional groups.

The scale and complexity of RM, involving as it does people across the organisation, emphasises the importance of planning change.   Indeed, the implementation of RM is in significant measure about planned change.   Yet RM involves two different types of change: and while one is planned, the other is unplanned, or organic (Burns and Stalker, 1966).   The first consists of those developments which can be clearly specified and timetabled, and managed separately from on-going processes (see Box 3.13).   At the sites these were typically organised as distinct sub-projects, each concerned with a particular aspect of RM, co-ordinated by a project manager and team.   As the implementation progressed, the planned changes incorporated some (but never all) aspects of organisation development.   The second type of change initially involves clarifying the overall objectives for implementation, and working out how they might be achieved, either through planned or organic change.   Then, crucially, as change begins to occur those involved have to rethink roles and processes continuously: organic change is organisation-wide, and events occurring in one part of the organisation may ripple through to affect others.

There is a great deal of interplay between the planned and organic processes, and it is this which gives RM both its complexity and its dynamism.   With RM being experimental in nature, the organic element was strong, particularly in the early stages, but as the Initiative progressed more and more elements were brought into the formal planning process.   Prototyping approaches were linked to formal planning processes (Checkland, 1988; Rowen, 1990).   Yet it seems that there must remain a substantial and important organic element which leads to a need for continuous review of all plans for RM.

One of the key questions about the implementation concerns how the two major strands distinguished in this chapter, information and organisation and structure, fit together to form a single, coherent entity which is RM.   In general terms, the strands are linked by two concepts, communication and control (Checkland, 1988).   The result of the organisation development processes and the adoption of formal sub-unit structures is that new lines of communication across professional and departmental boundaries are established.   A distinctive feature of the structures, perhaps most evident at sub-unit level, is that the nature of monitoring and decision making changes, with the involvement of members of different staff groups meaning that a wide range of knowledge and information can be fed in to management processes.   These new processes are centrally concerned with control of resources.

A principal purpose of the computer systems is to facilitate communication by providing data for planning, monitoring and evaluation of services.   In practice, the sites reached a point where new lines of communication had been opened up, but their information systems had not yet reached the point where they were an integral

Box 3.13 The RM project planning process

1   Unit staff collaborate in
     clarifying and setting objectives.

2   Project team develops
     project plan.

3   Resources allocated to project.

4   Project plan implemented
     by project team.

5   Progress monitored by project
     manager and team.

6   Progress evaluated by project
     team and unit.

part of these lines of communication. Similarly, the control of resources involved service providers, but the principal sources of data were the pre-existing budgeting systems. New systems were beginning to be used, but the various systems implemented had not yet been integrated to the extent originally envisaged by the sites.

There are two issues which merit further examination in the light of the experiences of the sites. First, there appears to be an underlying theme which goes some way towards explaining the variety of experiences observed. There are several possible purposes for implementing a large centralised database such as the RM database: to support service planning, improve control of resource use, facilitate review of clinical work, support research projects, and so on (Galliers, 1987). In principle, at least, the data in the database can be used for any of these purposes, since it contains detailed individual patient data which can be manipulated in a variety of ways. At the sites, two uses have been most important: control of resource use and review of care. In general, those at the sites involved in the design of the RM databases perceived them as tools for better control of resource use, and they were initially designed to support unit or sub-unit management. This did not exclude the possibility that they would also be used more widely for review of care processes, but this would be dealt with later. Only Huddersfield started out with an explicit focus on review of clinical work rather than control of resource use, a point also noted by Coombs *et al.* (1990).

This opposition of control and review may explain why many service providers did not show any interest in using available data: they perceived the systems as instruments of control. Others, in contrast, were sanguine about the issue of control or simply perceived the value of data for review of their own work, and so made use of it.

Looking at the same issues on a wider scale, there have also been discussions about what data units and districts should receive from sub-units. Confidentiality is an important issue here, with the discussions increasingly coloured by perceived data requirements for contracting. This issue remains to be resolved.

The second issue raised by the RM implementation strategies adopted by the sites concerns the initial concentration on in-patient activity data. The reasons for this were pragmatic, having their origins in perceived shortcomings of MB computer systems, and in the assumption that passing operational data concerning in-patients to RM databases would be achieved fairly quickly. But since progress has been slower than expected, it is prudent to consider the value of the data from the new computer systems that the sites have available. The judgements of managers and service providers at the sites were highly variable, as noted above, suggesting that no clear answer has yet emerged.

Box 3.14 Current status of RM implementation at the six sites, autumn 1990
(◨ = partial: some systems accurate and complete; ■ = implemented; □ = not yet implemented)

Component	Benchmark	Arrowe Park	Freeman	Guy's	Huddersfield	Pilgrim	Royal Hampshire
Operational system-RM database links	Maximal accuracy/completeness for in-patients	□	◨	◨	■	◨	◨
	Business Managers obtain most data direct from computer systems or computer printouts	□	■	■	■	□	□
Coding	Coders formally attached to specialties	■	■	□	■	■	■
Care profiles	Nursing profiles developed	■	■	■	■	■	■
	Consultant profiles developed	□	□	□	■	□	□
Computerised ward nursing dependency/workload systems	Installed across hospital	□	□	■	■	■	■
Budgets	Case mix costs routinely available to sub-units	□	□	□	□	□	□
	Management budgets held at sub-unit level	■	■	■	■	■	■
Organisation	Unit-wide sub-unit management structure	■	■	■	■	□	■

Obviously, the value of the new data was limited principally to discussions of in-patient activity. Unit and sub-unit level consideration of activity elsewhere in the hospital was not supported by detailed data on activities, or the costs of those activities. In retrospect, some sites felt they might have started elsewhere: Huddersfield with nursing, for example, which would both have provided data on a major area of resource use and perhaps drawn nurses earlier into involvement with other disciplines. Additionally, some consultants felt that an earlier emphasis on out-patient data would have been preferable. In this they are supported by the Review, which appears to place particular emphasis on out-patient data.

CONCLUSION

RM was in practice more experimental than predictable at the sites, with some major elements still under development after four years. RM was a far larger undertaking than anyone initially imagined, in respect of both the information system implementation and organisation development. This being the case, it is not surprising that the original estimate of two years for implementation was greatly exceeded, but the result was that the various elements of RM were not yet integrated into a whole. Nevertheless, sites learned a great deal about planning and managing large projects, made considerable progress with implementation of new information systems, and underwent major organisation development, exemplified by the widespread adoption of new unit and sub-unit management structures. Box 3.14 summarises the status of the sites in the autumn of 1990.

Chapter 4

THE RM PROCESS

INTRODUCTION

The initial guidance on RM (DHSS, 1986a) hinted at the importance of process through the involvement of service providers, together with managers, in making informed choices regarding the application of resources. Our Interim Report to the Department of Health elaborated on this (Buxton *et al.*, 1989), suggesting that RM should be thought of as a dynamic process of management, rather than as a single discrete activity. And further, that this process employed a traditional and familiar management cycle.

This chapter commences by explaining the nature of this RM process as we conceptualised it, and then examines its application as we have observed it in the six sites. This examination is broken down into three distinct levels, namely that of: the individual work set; individuals grouped in sub-units organised around discrete services; and, the hospital unit as a whole. Since different aspects of the process are more or less developed at the different sites, the examination first concentrates upon general aspects of the application of the RM process across all six sites. This is undertaken in terms of five inter-related elements that appeared to be crucial in determining engagement with the RM process at all of the three levels within a unit organisation. These comprise:

■ commitment by the relevant personnel at each level;

■ devolution of authority to meaningfully engage in the process at each level;

■ collaboration within and between disciplines in securing the objectives of RM;

■ means for management to occur, particularly in terms of organisation structure and provision of information (these represent resource costs for RM and are further discussed in Chapter 5);

■ the focus of the local RM strategy.

Naturally these five elements operate in different ways between the three organisational levels and in different situations. A brief section of the chapter then considers the linkages between the three levels, which, in our judgement, are crucial to the success of the RM process. The chapter concludes with some tentative and general assessments of the application of the RM process at the six sites.

THE NATURE OF THE PROCESS

The RM process, with its five main steps is depicted in Box 4.1. Although the cycle is a familiar management tool, it is worth stressing the innovatory features which were less obvious but clearly crucial to its success:

- the process had to involve those service providers who actually committed resources in patient care. This certainly included the doctors and nurses, a target of RM since its inception, but also paramedics and managers of support services. But in so far as RM necessitated drawing the service providers into a dynamic management process, so the space for their involvement had to be made by the general managers and senior and middle ranking functional managers *not* directly involved in committing resources to patients, standing back; changing their role to facilitation and monitoring rather than direction. So RM entailed a 'bottom-up' as well as the more familiar 'top-down' view of decision-making, and thus represented an enormous cultural change to both sets of participant;

- the process would only move if service providers were given ready access to information that defined the resources that were available and related these to the activities performed in patient care. And if such information was to be made available, it required the service providers devoting more time and attention to both its provision and interpretation than had been the case hitherto;

- if the process gave service providers increased authority to manage resources for patient care, so it also required them to be accountable for their use. This pointed towards new organisational arrangements below the level of the unit, which usually marked the lowest level for general management in hospitals. The clinical directorate is perhaps the best known sub-unit structure claimed to facilitate the implementation of RM, but the general point is that RM required changes in the traditional organisation of specialties, departments and wards to reflect the new properties of authority and accountability. It also brought new roles into the organisation. In the case of RM project team leaders and project managers the new roles were obvious. But the latter were temporary requirements. The new permanent roles, such as clinical directors, clinical heads of department, chairmen of user groups, business managers and nurse managers, were less evident but vitally important in the long-term.

Our Interim Report also stressed that one of the difficulties in evaluating RM was that it was being implemented alongside existing management systems, which had to respond to other influences than RM. In this context we drew attention to an impressive list of changes inherited from past initiatives, ranging from Griffiths in

Box 4.1 The RM process

1   Service providers collaborate in setting objectives, priorities and plans.

2   Resources are allocated to service providers to achieve agreed priorities.

3   Service providers exercise responsibility for managing the resources they commit.

4   Service provision and resource use are regularly monitored.

5   The value of the service provided is reviewed.

1983 to the NHS Review in 1989. If in June 1989 the latter already represented a change in the weather for the operation of the NHS, by December 1990 it had become a change of climate. But if the RM process was to become part of the normal on-going management processes of the NHS, it could not remain immune from what represents the most potentially far reaching changes to the health service since 1948. The arrangement imposed for medical audit, to take one example, cannot help but effect the way in which clinicians monitor and evaluate their use of resources. The requirements of the provider role, to take another, will condition how services are planned and the resources available to service providers.

Whilst not elaborating the idea, the Interim Report suggested that the RM process operates simultaneously at different levels within the unit. (These are depicted in Box 4.2).

- Level 1 - the individual work set. A single clinical firm or a ward could apply the RM process to their own activities; defining their objectives and priorities, allocating the resources available to them accordingly, managing the application of these resources, monitoring their use and evaluating the services provided. Clearly individual objectives and priorities are dependent upon judgements of value made by those who are accountable for deploying resources at higher levels within the unit. The latter, too, are likely to have their own means for monitoring resource use and evaluating service provision.

- Level 2 - the sub-unit. A specialty, a clinical department or a directorate, or a group of wards performing a common function could apply the RM process to their collective activities. The tasks are to decide priorities and then direct and manage resources accordingly. This can never be easy. On the one hand, members of the sub-unit are likely to be restricted in their activities by the decisions and judgements of the resource providers at higher levels in the unit. On the other, they are likely to be equally restricted by the interests and preferences of their individual members. Thus to a greater or lesser extent the RM process at sub-unit level operates through a mixture of consensus and direction.

- Level 3 - the unit. The unit as a whole can engage in the RM process, providing the interface between general management, with its comprehensive accountability for unit performance and development, and the more specific interests of the service providers. The involvement of the latter will have to be structured by representative mechanisms and/or the managerial hierarchy, to both clarify responsibilities and to prevent the service providers from swamping the process. The task is the same, although exercised on a larger scale, as that at sub-unit level; agreeing priorities and then allocating and managing resources in order that

Box 4.2 Levels of the RM process

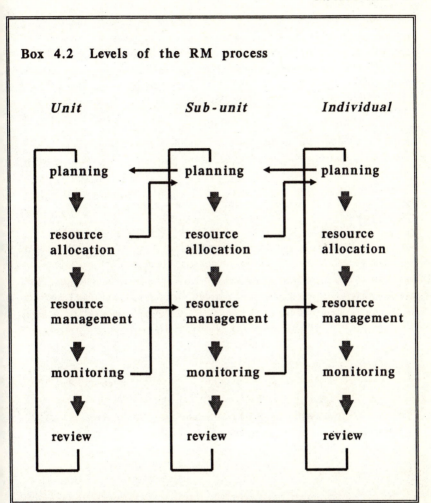

they are realised. Of course as well as being influenced by the wishes of coalitions of service providers, powerful baronies indeed, unit objectives and priorities are similarly subject to the decisions of resource providers at higher levels, who will also engage in monitoring the way in which the unit is applying its resources and evaluating the services it provides. By separating purchasers and providers, however, the proposals in the NHS Review radically change the ground rules by which both resources are allocated and services evaluated.

If the earlier definition of RM as involving bottom-up decision-making holds true, it might be expected that the RM process is an ascending and descending spiral. In the ascendent mode the objectives and priorities made as part of the individual process contribute to those made by the sub-unit, and the objectives and priorities of the sub-unit in turn contribute to the unit process. In the descendent mode the creation of plans and allocation of resources made at unit level prescribes, facilitates and supports the RM process at sub-unit level, which in turn influences the process at the individual level through its own planning and budgetary activities. Similarly the results of unit monitoring of services impacts on the discretion allowed to sub-units in managing their resources, and likewise for sub-units and individual work sets. Our observations suggest that nowhere does the RM process yet work as smoothly as the ideal sketched above. None the less Box 4.3 illustrates how the creation of unit objectives in one of the six sites brings together both higher level (district) and lower level (directorates) objectives. Recognising that the RM process does have to move between different levels helps to illuminate some of the tensions and strains that occur. The character of RM strikes differently at the individual, sub-unit and unit levels. The examination of the application of the RM process commences with the former.

RM AT THE INDIVIDUAL LEVEL

The extent to which service providers engaged with the RM process as individuals or as members of an individual work set such as a clinical firm or nursing ward, varied enormously both within and between sites.

In one sense, of course, many individuals saw themselves as intuitively engaging in the RM process. A consultant or a ward sister had to think about the work to be done, use resources such as time, beds, junior staff and drugs to best effect, keep an eye on how things were going and modify the service if this appeared necessary. But this approach is predominately reactive and *ad hoc*, shaped by the workload that presents itself, using resources determined by others, allocated accordingly to other priorities and managed by other specialist staff. If it is anything, the RM process sketched out in Box 4.4 is proactive, with individuals determining the pattern of work

Box 4.3   Origin of unit objectives

'The District Health Authority has set a number of objectives for the unit to achieve during 1989-90. These include:

monitoring and reduction of waiting lists;

realisation of benefits from the Hospital Information System;

extension of existing quality initiatives;

extension of Individual Performance Review down into the unit;

provision of a district policy statement on out-patient and in-patient waiting times.

The unit has absorbed and addressed these in this plan, as has each of the clinical directorates in its own statement of intentions for the five-year period. With regard to the policy statement on waiting times, however, the feasibility of producing a meaningful statement for the unit as a whole has been debated with individual clinical directors and at the Management Board. The clear consensus is that a specific statement must be made by each directorate; each directorate is therefore in the process of constructing its statement, and not all are presently available.

Furthermore, the unit has augmented the objectives set by the district by adding its own corporate objectives to the range of tasks it plans to achieve during the period. It has also incorporated *aims*: those areas where the *direction* of change is clearly set, but where the *pace* of change is not prescribed. These aims are included in the 1989-90 objectives as part of the whole five-year look since in all cases we intend to *commence* the task in the first year.

The principle, therefore, of the hierarchy of objectives - where each successive layer of the organisation absorbs the objectives it receives from above and adds in its own - is established in this plan, and fundamental to its implementation. clinical directorates' own plans acknowledge this principle'.

(Unit Business Plan, 1989)

Box 4.4   The RM process at the individual level

1   Individual consultant, ward sister or paramedical senior officer sets objectives, priorities and plans.

2   Resources are allocated to individuals to achieve agreed priorities.

3   Individuals exercise responsibility for managing the allocated resources.

4   Individuals monitor service provision and resource use.

5   Individuals review the value of the service provided.

they consider necessary and manipulating the available resources to achieve the most effective results.

The five inter-related elements that are relevant in determining the extent to which individuals participated in the RM process are set out in Box 4.5 and discussed below.

■ *A commitment to take on a proactive role in managing resources.* Throughout the evaluation, in all six sites, the main attraction of RM to service providers was the possibility that a more proactive role in managing resources could result in a better service to patients. Commitment by individuals occupying key decision-making positions, such as consultants and ward sisters, was crucial. In the event, commitment varied. RM had its champions and its assailants, although many, perhaps most, service providers remained uncommitted one way or the other. Perhaps RM would go away!

■ *Devolution of authority to the service providers.* This was necessary in order that they could manage their own resources to the best effect. This was hedged with difficulties in that individuals had to take account of existing demands and priorities set by higher levels. There is also the problem that one individual's work related with many others. Despite the traditional accusations of professional power, the scope for individual decision in the NHS is fairly limited. Only in two sites, for example, were nursing budgets said to be devolved to ward sisters, and even then practice apparently varied between sub-units. Devolution of budgetary authority was seen by many individual participants as vital if they were to take responsibility for managing resources but even when individual service providers held budgets, they were frequently described as notional rather than real, in that they were treated as a retrospective means of monitoring activities and the individual concerned was allowed little discretion to decide between different courses of action. Not surprisingly, there was little incentive for change.

■ *Collaboration with other disciplines.* If individual service providers are going to exercise a more proactive role in respect of their activities, they must, as suggested above, pay some regard to each other. A change in priorities by a surgical firm can have significant implications for the demand for theatre time, for the demand on other firms, for drugs, for nursing manpower, for physiotherapy, and so on. And because the provision of better quality care includes the conscious and responsible management of resources, so individual service providers have to engage in a dialogue with the managers who control their allocation. This may be through the sub-unit or via sub-unit based roles, if these exist and are part of the resource allocation process, or it may require direct negotiations with the unit general manager and functional heads of department.

Box 4.5   Participation of individual service providers in the RM process is encouraged if:

■   individuals are committed

    (need for perceived incentives)

■   individuals have devolved authority

    (need for perceived freedom of action)

■   individuals are prepared to collaborate with other disciplines

    (need for dialogue with colleagues and with unit/sub-unit managers)

■   individuals are supported in their management tasks

    (need for information and help with management activities)

■   RM strategy emphasises individual participation

    (need to formalise processes for individual participation in decision-making and provide information that meets individual requirements)

■ *The means for individuals to manage their resources.* These include:

Information regarding resources available, activities performed and their resource costs. Throughout the period of our study, case mix data was in the process of development and introduction. The development of medical audit also provided a stimulus for consultants to collect and interpret data. Information for individuals to engage in management does not have to be computerised, although computerisation may give important advantages in terms of speed, volume, scope and ease of manipulation. As the RM Initiative developed, computer based information systems were being extended and data made available to individuals.

Assistance. Individuals required assistance for the analysis and interpretation of the available information. RM project staff and/or business managers provided the main source of assistance, often as part of their monitoring role on behalf of the sub-unit.

Time. A frequent complaint was that the immediate effect of a process intended to benefit patient care, was less time available for patients. But complainants also generally expected this to be a temporary 'learning' phenomenon, and that nurses, for example, would actually have more time at the patients bedside when they had become familiar with the computers. And even if there was less time available for direct patient care, some suggested that the quality of that care should be improved because the service providers had greater knowledge of the resources that could be applied and of their implications. Perhaps individuals quickly forgot the time taken up pursuing the management of resources across hospitals before RM was introduced.

■ *The local RM strategy.* The sites, themselves, varied in the extent to which they focused on individual participation in the RM process as against participation at the sub-unit or unit levels, and whether they favoured a 'softly softly' approach, allowing individuals some leeway in how and when they became part of RM, or pursued a more directive strategy. Relevant considerations included:

Whether or not there was a directorate structure. In the absence of a directorate structure at the sub-unit level, the RM process perforce relied more upon individual participation. However, the involvement of a sub-unit in RM also encouraged and formalised individual participation.

The extent to which information systems had been developed in response to the requirements of individual service providers.

All the sites: had their share of individuals opposed to RM; placed limitations on what individuals could or couldn't do; had gaps in the information available and the support that could be given to the service providers; were moving towards some form of sub-unit structure and developing their information systems to meet the needs of general managers as well as service providers. But by the same token all six sites met the criteria for encouraging participation partially, and offered some encouragement to individuals to engage in RM. This was an early characteristic of the development of RM at Huddersfield Royal Infirmary (and later at Arrowe Park). One of the main strategies in gaining support from the service providers for RM was through the development of a RM database that enabled consultants to obtain episode data on their own patients and to define their own clinical care profiles. This encouraged them to take responsibility for monitoring the quantity and quality of patient care and to consider developing different patterns of care in discussion with management. The subsequent creation of Clinical User Groups provided a forum for aggregating and prioritising service providers' opinions at the sub-unit level, without moving to the formality and authority of a clinical directorate.

I am now more aware of the financial requirements within my ward. Also there is more information to the other ward staff. Quality of care delivered and work carried out is now more in question, which makes staff more responsible.

Ward Sister

RM AT THE SUB-UNIT LEVEL

If RM does imply a move towards a 'bottom-up' approach to decision-making, some mechanism nearer to the individuals than the unit would be helpful for aggregating and prioritising the preferences and performance of individual service providers, as well as for supplying a focus of accountability for the application and management of resources. The role of the sub-unit in the RM process is suggested in Box 4.6.

As with the previous section, we briefly discuss those inter-related factors that appear important in explaining the engagement of sub-units with RM. These are depicted in Box 4.7.

■ *Commitment to the sub-unit.* Although embryo sub-unit structures are a traditional feature of the NHS, the RM process is different in requiring one common sub-unit that subsumes and integrates the work of all the service

Box 4.6 The RM process at the sub-unit level

1 Consultants and senior nursing and paramedical staff in the sub-unit set objectives, priorities and plans.

2 Resources are allocated to the Head of sub-unit to achieve agreed priorities. Resources may be further devolved to individuals or groups.

3 Head of sub-unit, together with individuals or groups, exercises responsibility for managing the allocated resources.

4 Head of sub-unit, together with individuals and groups, monitors service provision and resource use.

5 Head, individuals and groups review the value of the service provided.

Box 4.7   Participation of sub-units within the RM process is encouraged if:

- individuals are committed

    (need to perceive an incentive in collective values)

- sub-unit has developed authority

    (need for perceived freedom of collective action)

- members of the sub-unit are able to collaborate

    (need for mechanisms to promote collective participation in RM process)

- sub-unit managers are supported in their work

    (need for information and for specialist managerial roles)

- RM strategy emphasises sub-unit organisation

    (need for information and implementation strategy that are appropriate to sub-unit structure and processes) providers, rather than consisting of a number of separate specialty groupings and separately managed disciplines. Its very existence signifies that its members accept the need to accommodate the values and interests of colleagues and other disciplines. Commitment would appear to require meaningful collaboration, which is discussed below. Respondents claimed that sub-units, particularly those formally organised as directorates with heads who exercised accountability for, and authority over, the work of other members, did develop a strong identity and a 'brand loyalty' among their staff.

■ *Devolution of authority to the sub-unit.* This too encourages commitment. It is certainly a requirement of the RM process but the extent to which it occurs varies both between sites and within sites according to the circumstances that arise. Those sub-units with which we worked closely, demonstrated an increasing inclination to determine their own objectives and to then direct the available resources accordingly, preserving one service at the expense of others or deciding where additional efforts were required. All three sites with clinical directorates claimed that two-thirds to three-quarters of total unit resources were managed by the directorates, although the degree of freedom to significantly alter expenditure patterns may be limited by the need to gain approval from the unit level, which must consider wider hospital, disciplinary and community interests.

Sub-units experience the same problems in relation to devolution as does the individual service provider, having to take account of existing demands and of the priorities set both by higher levels and by individuals in their own work, while remaining aware of the inter-relationship with other sub-units. Greater freedom for one may only be gained at the expense of another.

■ *Collaboration between disciplines.* At sub-unit level the RM process requires the consultants, as the main resource users, to work out a consensus to shape their practice to the available resources, to agree common priorities and to adapt their own work as a result of collective monitoring and service review. For other hierarchically managed disciplines it means putting operational service requirements on a par with, or above, specialised professional interests. And the sub-unit as a whole has to contribute its vision to help shape wider unit objectives, and negotiate the supply of resources with unit managers.

Our respondents differed in their perceptions as to the extent to which collaboration, even in its weaker informing and advisory modes, was a reality. Certainly some, and from different disciplines, saw the increase in multi-disciplinary working as one of the chief benefits of RM. But others saw that status differentials lingered, both within and between disciplines. The nursing voice, for example, was now represented by one specialty manager and was not seen as carrying the same weight as that of the consultants.

Communication was further hampered by information strategies which had been developed with the requirements of single disciplines in mind.

Clinical freedom in its old sense, is dead - but long live clinical responsibility based on accurate information and informed opinion.

A. Brooks, Consultant Physician
British Medical Journal, 1990

An example of collaboration between consultants in a directorate in reviewing their collective activities and shaping their practice is given in Box 4.8. This illustrates how a clinical director can use information as a basis for discussing future service production, as well as the existence of multiple and conflicting views as to the appropriate course of action.

Sub-units deliberately set up processes to formalise and foster collaboration. These were seen as having two benefits: improved working relationships, through providing access to information and the opportunity to participate in reaching decisions; and, improved patient care, through the ability to focus attention on related services. In many cases these processes had existed before but were frequently informal and depended upon individual interest and style. Examples include: regular weekly business meetings between heads and business and nurse managers; regular monthly meetings between the consultant members; and, general meetings that were open to all staff which, although hardly forums for joint management, at least provided information on plans and priorities and their progress.

Increase in meetings - approximately two per week. Less time to support colleagues and for patients.

Ward Sister

In our survey (see Appendix 1) 59 per cent of nurses felt that since RM had been introduced relationships with consultants had improved. However other respondents interviewed over the course of the research were less confident that the creation of a sub-unit changed anything. Collaboration, as always, depended upon individual personalities.

Box 4.8 Consultants meeting in a directorate - October 1989

Present: clinical director, four other consultants, senior registrar, business
    manager, researcher

Item - varicose veins

The clinical director produced information regarding the monthly additions to the
waiting lists for both in-patients and day patients. He and a second consultant
agreed to reduce the day case waiting list by treating two or three extra cases each
month. The clinical director then proposed reducing the in-patient list by creating
a special waiting list of patients who were prepared to be admitted at short notice
if there was a gap in theatre lists. The third consultant argued that this would not
help. You could not solve problems by *ad hoc* measures, filling a vacant slot. It
was necessary to draw up plans to take three extra in-patient admissions each
month. The second consultant said that he could not participate in this. The
third and fourth consultants felt that they could, although the latter wondered if
the financial position meant that they could reduce varicose vein cases? The
clinical director argued that hopefully the financial crisis (which he was coming to
later) was a short term problem, whereas reducing the waiting list was a matter of
principle. The second consultant wondered if a registrars' varicose vein list could
be treated on Monday mornings when there was a free theatre session? The
clinical director agreed to investigate and check if an anaesthetist was available.
The fifth consultant warned that the theatre was used for teaching purposes at this
time and was not, in fact, available. The clinical director would investigate. The
third consultant stressed that reducing the waiting list was a priority. The fifth
consultant proposed adopting 'a blitz strategy' to get the waiting list down to an
acceptable level. He was supported by the third consultant who also suggested the
some of the figures relating to varicose vein operations were wrong. The clinical
director asked the business manager to check the figures. The fourth consultant
reminded the meeting that 'a blitz' on the waiting list would require additional
funds. The clinical director agreed to investigate the possibility of additional
finance from the current central government initiative being available.

■ *The means for sub-unit management.* These included:

> *Provision of information.* Members, particularly managers and/or leaders,
> require to be aware of the activities being performed and how resources are
> being applied. One frequent criticism was that the managers and leaders had
> access to information that was not shared among all the other members. In
> the sub-units we observed closely, practice varied according to: the presence
> or absence of a policy on access to data; and, the wishes of the head of the
> sub-unit. For example, in one site which had a policy on data access, one
> sub-unit was distributing activity data to its members; while because of doubts
> to its accuracy, another sub-unit restricted circulation of the data to the head
> and his immediate managers.

I personally receive very little directly relevant information. Clinical
leaders and directorates do not distribute it, except in very general terms.

Consultant

> *Provision of management.* Even if all the members do their share, the task of
> managing resources on behalf of the sub-unit requires some committed time.
> It cannot be done as an extension of the professional role, and calls for
> definitive skills, both politically and administrative, that professionals do not
> necessarily possess. Indeed as discussed earlier, at the sub-unit level the
> chairman or head, the business manager and the nurse manager will all be
> engaged in specialist management work. But this does not necessarily imply
> that the management has become an increased burden. It is probably more
> visible with RM but many of the tasks had to be performed before the
> initiative, although not necessarily by the same people, nor at the sub-unit
> level, nor were they necessarily explicit. Supporters of RM would claim that
> it has resulted in more explicit and more purposive management.

■ *The local RM strategy.* Initially the sites appeared to diverge sharply as to whether
RM was best approached from the standpoint of a strong organisational structure,
which meant in fact gearing information requirements and planning
implementation to the structures and processes of the sub-units, or to approach
RM from strong data provision, which meant giving more emphasis to the
requirements of individual managers and service providers. Three sites took the
former path, three the latter. The choice partly reflected the preferences of those

who were charged with implementing RM and was partly explained by what was already in place, itself a product of earlier processes and the predominant local culture. Both Guy's and the Royal Hampshire County Hospital had a directorate structure in place, whereas Freeman and Pilgrim commenced the experiment with strong and committed unit management.

As was the case with the individual level of RM process, the criteria that encourage participation in sub-unit organisation were all present to a limited extent. Not surprisingly they were more prominent in those hospitals which chose to emphasise sub-unit organisation from the outset than in those that emphasised other priorities. But in all cases there was commitment, sometimes considerable, to working collectively as a sub-unit; after all the other members were colleagues with whom some degree of informal working would be necessary whatever the arrangements. Authority to manage resources had been devolved, although not always sufficiently to make sub-units feel that they were controlling their own destiny, and not necessarily in a consistent manner. Devolution of budgetary responsibility to sub-units appeared crucial in this context. By 1991 this is to be expected to be the case in all six sites. It was also crucial that the sub-units received support in the task of managing their resources, both in terms of information supply and appropriately skilled bodies. Over the last three years data has increasingly been focused at the sub-unit level but complaints were made that activity and costing data was still unavailable and that some disciplines were far better served than others. It had also become realised that the scale of involvement in the RM process at the sub-unit level required the management of services to be bolstered with specialist support. Such support was not regarded as an extravagance and all the sites treated it as an important priority, providing it in some cases as a central service to sub-units but more usually as a devolved function. RM implementation strategies, always balancing between developing the computer technology and the human processes, all, sooner or later, gave attention to sub-unit organisation.

Detailed observation of sub-units in action at Freeman and the Royal Hampshire County Hospital provided examples of the RM process: of frank exchange of viewpoints between different disciplines and a greater understanding of others concerns as a result; of colleagues being able to discuss each others workload and agree changes to accommodate new demands and alterations in the available resources; of agreement on what does and does not represent a priority; and, of collective agreement on improved ways of managing resources. But there have also been examples where issues have proved difficult, or too sensitive, to resolve, and have become long running agenda items, or where the sub-unit's freedom has been abruptly curtailed by decisions taken elsewhere.

> I feel no change has occurred in what actually happens on the shop floor. The mechanisms within the system have changed but the end result has produced nothing dissimilar from 'the old days'. We all have plenty of clinical energy but no money, and RM has not altered that.
>
> Consultant

RM AT THE UNIT LEVEL

Since the RM experiment was applied to six acute hospital units, the existence of some form or other of unit organisation was obviously one of the few common factors in all the sites participating in the RM experiment. Thus the unit, embodied in the role of its general manager, already had an identity in terms of management process. Indeed, in so far as units had to prioritise and plan, allocate resources, ensure that these were managed and monitor their application, they already engaged in something like the RM process. But similarities cannot be extended too far. Traditional unit management left little room for resources to be managed by the service providers, and as a result resources were allocated from above more than managed. The RM process at unit level as depicted in Box 4.9 is about creating, supporting and maintaining processes further down the organisation, and aggregating and deciding between service strategies. In other words, in one respect the RM process reverses traditional management practices between unit and individual levels, and in consequence unit management is required to be more reactive and less directive than has had to be the case hitherto.

Units, of course, were never completely free agents. Although they had been strengthened by recent policies to move authority and identification of service accountability closer to the patient, they had been created by districts, were accountable to districts, resourced by districts and required to recognise district priorities. And, looking in the other direction, they were also restricted by the actions of the service providers, who, individually or collectively, determined service delivery.

This section continues the previous form of analysis by briefly sketching the five inter-related factors that appear crucial in determining unit engagement with the RM process. These are depicted in Box 4.10.

■ *Unit commitment to the RM process.* Unit commitment was crucial to RM for a number of fairly obvious reasons. First, the investment of time and money in RM required the sanction of senior officers at the unit level, as did the development of new procedures. Second, their efforts and expertise were needed to get RM

Box 4.9   The RM process at the unit level

1   Unit managers and service heads/
    representatives set ojectives,
    priorities and plans.

2   Resources are allocated to the
    unit to achieve agreed priorities.

3   Unit managers exercise responsibility
    for managing resources. Some is
    devolved to service providers, the
    remainder stays under unit control.

4   Unit managers monitor service
    provision and resource use.

5   Unit managers engage with service
    heads/representatives in reviewing
    the value of the service provided.

Box 4.10   Participation of units within the RM process is encouraged if:

- unit managers are committed

    (need to perceive benefits for the unit and/or for tasks of management)

- unit has devolved authority

    (need to maximise ability to meet demands)

- unit managers are prepared to collaborate with service providers

    (need for mechanisms to include service providers in unit processes)

- unit management is supported in its work

    (need for accurate information regarding service provision)

- RM strategy emphasises unit organisation

    (need for information and implementation strategy that provides for unit ownership and relates RM to unit management processes)

'off the ground'. Staff at unit level possessed key skills in such areas as information provision, costing, planning and day to day management of resources. These skills were required by the service providers if they were to engage in RM. Third, if RM was to make any impact on the organisation, it had to influence the essential unit management and planning procedures.

Our observation was that unit commitment was variable. Where it was present it proved a strong driving force to the whole RM process; where it was absent RM suffered or perforce had to rely on inputs from other levels, such as committed service providers or from district roles.

Commitment partly reflected personal viewpoints as to the value or 'faddishness' of RM, it also reflected whether RM had been seen as an imposition on the unit from elsewhere. The relationship between the unit and higher authorities was crucial. In some cases RM, at least initially, was seen as a district policy. In many cases aspects of district and regional policies were seen as working to help or hinder aspects of RM. For the most part unit managers welcomed RM as helping them to do a better job, in so far as it would give them more effective control over resources and thereby enable better services to be provided to patients. But occupying the interface between the organisation delivering services and the wider environment, unit managers have to react to many demands. As the experiment continued work on the NHS Review proposals meant that they were increasingly stretched and inevitably had less time to spare for RM, or began to see its contribution in new ways.

- *Devolution of authority to the unit.* In considering the implementation of the RM process at both the individual and sub-unit level, much was made of the unit's willingness or reluctance to devolve authority. When the focus shifts to the unit, so the potential barriers shift, and units prove dependent upon decisions made by higher levels, as well as by the willingness of those working at lower levels to accept responsibility. Districts and regions will have priorities that units are obliged to follow. The question of the extent to which districts were prepared to meet the costs of inflation was seen as particularly vexed. However, unit officers argued that RM, by enabling plans and priorities to be based on the resources required for defined activities, should work to strengthen units' independence. Their case for resources was stronger if it was made on an accurate assessment of what was required to meet local needs, rather than on history or hunch.

- *Collaboration between disciplines.* Unit managers have always had to work with and through their service providers. Their ability to manage their doctors and nurses has frequently been hard earned and a source of pride. But with RM all are engaged in management and as the involvement of service providers in management increases, so they are likely to seek a more formal and favoured role in unit processes. So, too, unit managers may prefer to work less through individual negotiations and charisma, although these are likely to remain important parts of the armoury, and seek more regular forms of collaboration. Thus sites with clinical directorates, which require service providers to take accountability for management of resources, all have the directors constituting the majority membership of unit management boards. This enables service providers to join with unit based managers in determining priorities, allocating resources and monitoring their application, and so blends unit processes with those of the sub-units. And as the RM experiment has proceeded, sites that were less enthusiastic for strong sub-unit structures have none the less also experienced demands to strengthen the mechanisms for providing clinical advice at the unit level.

It has been asserted that collaboration with the service providers is facilitated if the UGM or chairman of the Hospital Board is also a service provider. This has been the case throughout in three of our sites, for a short period in a fourth and has not occurred in the remaining two. It does not appear to be a necessary condition, although it may serve to allay initial fears.

■ *The means for engaging in the RM process.* Unit officers required information to aggregate and monitor the demands made by service providers. Information systems were developed to provide unit managers with data, as much as the service providers. Indeed much of the data is the same, although at unit level it is likely to be aggregated and not identifiable in terms of individual patient episodes. This, of course, has fuelled suspicions that information for higher management provides the *raison d'être* of RM, that in reality it is all about tighter resource controls. The reality appears to be that much of the information available to unit managers is a by-product of that available to the service providers. If it is accepted that unit managers are as concerned with quality of services as they are with controlling resources, this must be entirely appropriate. In any case, the emphasis on supplying activity data means that the development of costing has tended to lag behind other aspects of RM.

Provision of information has also necessitated setting up new roles to work with the service providers in collecting and disseminating information; interpreting their viewpoints and needs to unit level, and unit level viewpoints to the service providers.

■ *The local RM strategy.* In four sites from the six, those primarily responsible for implementing RM have always been located at the unit level, and in one of the two sites where this was not initially the case, it subsequently proved advantageous to make the change. Unit responsibility emphasised local ownership, visible evidence that RM was not being imposed by others, and also enabled a comprehensive strategy to be devised, drawing in different parts of the organisation and different disciplines. The extent to which responsibility for RM lay elsewhere, and no unit was wholly master of its own destiny, gave rise to problems, both in terms of project management and in terms of ownership of data; problems that were subsequently highlighted by the purchaser/provider distinction brought in by the NHS Review. On the other hand, if district and regions worked with units they could prove valuable sources of expertise for the development of RM, possessing skills in information services and financial analysis which units lacked, as well as sources of funding.

However there were also problems with this unit focus. Individuals involved in implementing RM frequently had to share this responsibility with other duties. Opinions varied as to how far this was a strength, in providing the individual concerned with an identity, keeping in touch with reality and helping integrate RM with other activities, or a weakness in terms of dilution of effort and distraction. The broad unit vision did not always appear aware of the complications and sensitivities existing at lower levels; and in so far as these were seen as objects whose activities had to be changed, the need for change at the unit level, itself, was perhaps neglected. If RM was to become part of the normal management processes, it had to be seen as relevant to those management processes that were the most obvious, and these tended to occur at unit level. Critics felt that all too often unit management processes were responding to other requirements and/or immediate convenience rather than adhering to the principles of the RM process. In this respect that attitude of the UGM to RM was crucial, carrying a symbolic value across the organisation.

Without unit involvement, RM is untenable. But there is a vast difference between encouraging others at lower levels to participate, as to a greater or lesser extent happened at all sites, and actively adapting unit processes and procedures to reflect, and encourage, the management of resources by the service providers. Where such adaptation occurred, it largely appeared as incremental and retrospective rather than concurrent with changes at lower levels. Arrowe Park was able to explicitly tie its structural re-organisation to the requirements of RM as, perhaps less dramatically, were Freeman and Huddersfield. The structural initiatives at both Guy's and Royal Hampshire that altered the power distribution in the respective units predated the official RM experiment. Unit managers differed in the extent to which they responded to RM with conviction, one at least displaying scepticism, and units, themselves, lacked in many respects the necessary freedom to respond positively to RM. As a breed, unit managers may feel more positive towards the new technology than many of the service providers but they, too, cannot use what is not available.

LINKAGES BETWEEN LEVELS

For the sake of simplicity the three levels engaged in the RM process have been largely treated as if they were separate strata. In actuality they present a contorted configuration: on some issues the levels are far apart and isolated, on others very close; on some issues one or two of the levels may not be engaged, on others they are all closely intertwined, with leadership switching from one to the other. The fact that the influence and role of the different levels is dynamic according to the circumstances and individuals involved in the RM process, reinforces the point made earlier regarding the importance of the linkages that exist between levels.

These linkages are of two kinds, processual and role and in either case they can be formal or informal. Box 4.11 indicates examples of the kind of linkages that we have observed between adjacent levels; that is between individual work sets and sub-units and between sub-units and units.

The examples, which are in no way exhaustive suggest that:

■ many of the linkages between levels in the RM process were in no way the product of RM. For example, UGMs and unit functional managers have always found it advisable to keep in touch with the service providers. UGMs and finance departments have sought to negotiate budgets with individual clinicians or specialties. Planning processes for a specialty or a discipline have usually attempted some aggregation of individual interests and priorities;

■ the informal linkages, as is always the case, may prove very important. A chance, or not chance, contact between a unit manager and a member of a sub-unit can lead to review and changes in the way in which resources are being managed.

Notwithstanding the two preceding points the RM process does appear to benefit from the development of formal linkages that were absent or less common in the past. These (starred in Box 4.11) include the following:

■ planning processes that explicitly focus on and aggregate the plans of lower levels;

■ planning processes that bring together the key individuals from lower levels, as in sub-unit staff or business meetings and in unit board, council or advisory meetings;

■ provision of trusted information that is relevant in reviewing the performance of adjacent levels, as in the contribution of individual activity to sub-unit

Box 4.11 Linkages between levels in the RM process

A. *Individual work sets and sub-units*

	Process	Role
Formal	Sub-unit business meetings (Head, Nurse Manager, Business Manager)* Sub-unit staff meetings* Specialty planning Audit meetings Information for review on individual or sub-unit performance*	Head of division/director* Nurse manager* Business manager* Specialty chair Other roles with designated sub-unit responsibilities*
Informal	Discussion or exchange of information between members of a sub-unit	Any member of the sub-unit

B. *Sub-units and units*

	Process	Role
Formal	Unit Board/Council* Service advisory committees Unit planning processes that involve sub-unit plans* Specialty budgeting Information for review on sub-unit or unit performance*	UGM Unit functional managers Heads of division/directors* Clinical representatives Nurse managers* Business managers*
Informal	Discussions or exchange of information between members of a unit	Any members of sub-unit or unit management

* Forms of linkage that have developed concurrently with RM

performance (or vice versa), or that of sub-units to unit performance (or vice versa);

■ existence of roles that can appreciate the perspective of different levels, such as business managers interpreting the sub-unit concerns to individuals and individual concerns to sub-unit managers, and heads of division fulfilling the same role between unit and sub-units;

■ the presence of a formal sub-unit structure which does, in itself, represent an important mechanism of linkage between individual work sets of service providers and the hospital unit. But, as has been said elsewhere, sites vary in the extent to which they see that sub-units are, first, necessary and, second, necessitate formal arrangements.

In general terms, throughout the period of the RM experiment all sites increased the mechanisms for linkage between the three levels. This must be possibly explained by other pressures on traditional mechanisms, such as those imposed by the NHS Review on UGMs and clinical representatives.

ADOPTION OF THE RM PROCESS

Comparisons are often misleading and RM is no exception to this. Rather than attempting to make a detailed comparison between the six sites regarding their application of the various steps and levels that comprise the RM process, a generalised comparison has been made, in a simplified format.

It should be stressed that this represents impressionistic qualitative judgements of progress over the whole period of the experiment, and may well have been overtaken by more recent events. It is also possible that the researchers have been too greatly influenced by those specialties that were studied in detail.

First, Box 4.12, summarises the extent to which the sites, collectively, have engaged significantly with the RM process. This suggests that:

■ Engagement by service providers in the RM process is stronger and certainly wider (although still by no means complete) where authority and accountability is focused on sub-units; that is where it is devolved from units and aggregated from individual work sets. This has been the case throughout the experiment at Guy's and Royal Hampshire and has been the first priority at Arrowe Park. Sub-unit management at Freeman and Huddersfield evolved more gradually over the experiment, stimulated finally by the demands of the post-review NHS.

■ It has proved easier to engage with prioritising and planning how services will be provided (step 1 of RM process), management of the available resources (step 3),

Box 4.12   Engagement with the RM process

1. Prioritising and planning
   by service providers.

   Yes, although more in terms
   of service products and
   activities than outcomes.

2. Resource allocation according
   to plans agreed with service
   providers.

   Slight, difficult to unlock
   historic allocations or avoid
   incremental decisions.

3. Management of resources by
   service providers.

   Yes, particularly at the sub-
   unit level. A major gain from
   RM.

4. Monitoring of services and
   resource use.

   Yes, although it has taken
   time to obtain accurate,
   relevant data.

5. Service evaluation

   Slight, hindered by lack of
   information and the absence
   of freedom and/or incentive
   to significantly alter service
   provision.

monitoring of services provided and resource use (step 4), perhaps because these elements offer the strongest attraction to either/or unit managers and service providers. Budgetary allocations (step 2) obstinately reflected historical principles, and/or financial crises, regardless of the service providers having created new priorities and plans. Service evaluation (step 5) where service performance is reviewed in the light of measures of outcome and/or services' success in meeting their objectives, was hindered both by lack of relevant information and by inability or unwillingness to make major changes to solve problems. But as service providers become more engaged with the other steps in the RM process, so they are likely to face pressures to formally review the value of their activities as a basis for planning, thereby closing the cycle.

Second, the main structural levels in the RM process emphasised by the various sites over the period of the experiment are shown in Box 4.13. All levels in all the sites could hardly avoid being involved with RM to a greater or lesser extent, but Box 4.13 indicates our judgement as to where the major emphasis were placed over the period of the experiment as a whole. Thus:

- Arrowe Park emphasised sub-unit management within the corporate unit framework;

- Freeman has led the RM process through active unit management, while developing sub-unit specialty management more gradually;

- Guy's emphasised sub-unit management, although unit management has latterly been perceived as increasing in influence;

- Huddersfield emphasised individual participation in the RM process within the unit management framework;

- Pilgrim was initially district led to get RM under way, but has worked to develop unit ownership;

- Royal Hampshire emphasised sub-unit management within the corporate unit framework.

For the most part the RM process has been unit driven. This reflects the way in which RM has been implemented in the sites and it is to be expected that the involvement of individual service providers will increase with greater exposure.

> People are thinking more about the care they are giving. Staff are also thinking in a more cost effective mode.
>
> Senior Staff Nurse

Box 4.13   Principal level of engagement with the RM process over the experiment - by site

Levels	Arrowe Park	Freeman	Guy's	Huddersfield	Pilgrim	Royal Hampshire
Individual				✓		
Sub-unit	✓	✓	✓			✓
Unit	✓	✓	✓	✓	✓	✓
District					✓	

CONCLUSION

The wide recognition of the value of the RM process and its increased application in all six sites over the period of the experiment, represents one of the most positive results of our evaluation.

The RM process is a necessary condition for achieving successful RM, and indeed it can be seen as becoming part and parcel of normal general management. This chapter has examined the factors that appear to help in implementing the process, while suggesting that these may look rather different from the perspective of the individual service providers, the group of individuals within the sub-unit and at the level of the unit as a whole. The first and last of these had clear, if not necessarily particularly compatible identities in the management process before RM. The implementation of RM has worked to give greater prominence to sub-units, and it could be suggested that both service providers and general managers find it easier for the former to engage in management through some formal grouping.

Discussion of implementation ties the RM process back to issues of the availability and scope of computer systems, to organisation structure and to training and development, which were discussed in the previous chapter. It appears as one of the paradoxes of RM that a process aimed at strengthening and widening decision-making by individual service providers, requires strong leadership from hospital managers if it is to get off the ground.

But achieving the RM process is a means to achieving the goals of RM, not, in itself, an end. And it is a means that, inevitably, carries resource costs. These issues are considered further in the succeeding chapters.

Chapter 5

THE RESOURCE REQUIREMENTS OF RM

INTRODUCTION

RM has effected many different aspects of activity at the sites, and the commitment of a range of different types of resource. The RM process involves the redistribution of existing resources within the sites, as well as the application of new resources from other sources and, furthermore, the resources are committed both to the initial implementation of RM and to support the on-going RM process. This Chapter considers the nature and scale of the different flows of resources.

There are two key issues to be considered in the identification and measurement of resources devoted to RM. The first of these is concerned with the perspective that should be adopted. Those parties which have provided resources to the sites may be primarily interested in how their resources were utilised: these include the Department of Health, regions, districts, computer suppliers and management consultants. This view is illustrated in Box 5.1, showing where resources originate. But decisions about where resources should be committed have been made by the six hospitals on the basis that the benefits of RM would be realised within the hospitals. Accordingly, the perspective adopted here is that of the hospitals, as shown in Box 5.2, with the focus on where resources are committed.

What is more, Boxes 5.1 and 5.2 both represent a static picture - a snapshot - of resource allocation. In practice, resources have been provided over time, and committed simultaneously to the RM projects and the RM process, as shown in Box 5.3. The RM projects comprise the implementation and development work which in large part take place separately from the on-going management and care processes. The RM process is part of the on-going management activity of the hospital, as outlined in Chapter 4. Box 5.4 illustrates the change in distribution of resources over time, with the arrow from the projects to the process representing the route whereby new developments are integrated into the process. Over time, the total resources committed to RM grow, and hence the sizes of the two boxes increases: they may be incorporated directly into the process, or into RM projects. The arrow flowing from the process to the projects represents unit resources allocated to the projects.

Eventually, RM should become fully integrated into the activities of the hospital. At this point, RM becomes inseparable from other activities, and it is impossible to assign costs specifically to RM. RM as a discrete project is complete, and no further resources are committed. However, if it is successful, RM as an on-going process

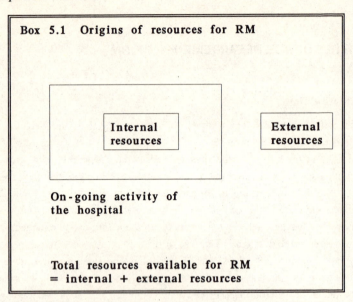

Box 5.1   Origins of resources for RM

Internal resources

External resources

On-going activity of the hospital

Total resources available for RM = internal + external resources

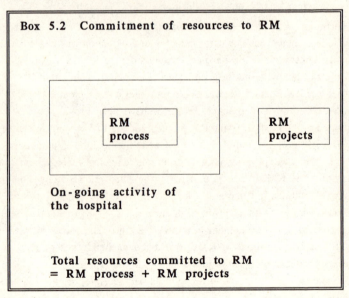

Box 5.2   Commitment of resources to RM

RM process

RM projects

On-going activity of the hospital

Total resources committed to RM = RM process + RM projects

Box 5.3   Flow of financial resources

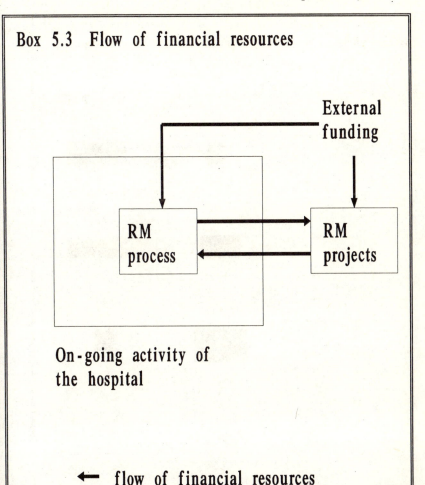

External funding

RM process

RM projects

On-going activity of the hospital

← flow of financial resources

Box 5.4   Relationship between RM process and projects over time

Time   On-going hospital activity   RM projects

t_1

t_2

t_3

t_4

───── > = flow of resources committed to RM

will not have an end point: it just keeps going and becomes indistinguishable from the management of the hospital. This is shown as time t_4 in Box 5.4. Of course, it is also possible that the RM projects and process fail to become integrated into the organisation. In this case the end state is not reached, the resources committed to the RM projects are only partially transferred into the process, and the process is still distinguishable from other hospital activities.

The second key issue concerns the conceptual distinction between investment in developing and implementing RM and the on-going running costs of a fully implemented project. The distinction is difficult to draw in practice in large, complex projects, where parts of a system can be fully implemented whilst others are still being developed. Certainly, this was the situation at the pilot sites, all of which were still implementing RM. It is possible to identify resources devoted to discrete RM projects, but more difficult to separate RM processes from other on-going activities.

A pragmatic approach has had to be taken to this problem. Estimates of the financial cost of the resources committed to RM projects and to sustain and develop RM processes are presented for the period of November 1986 to March 1990 (the beginning of the RM Initiative to the last complete financial year prior to the end of the evaluation). Taken together, these figures give a broad picture of the total investments made in RM during the period of the study. Additionally, indicative examples are given of the time spent by hospital staff on both the projects and the process.

The costs presented here reflect a number of important factors:

- that the sites started the national initiative at different points, both in terms of the development of their organisation structures and the number of departmental information systems implemented;

- that the sites have achieved different rates of progress in implementing various aspects of RM;

- and to some extent, that sites set different local objectives, some being broader and more complex than others.

The picture is further blurred by the concurrence of other important changes that also required resource inputs at the six sites during the period of the study. Principal among these was the NHS Review. Hospital staff devoted a great deal of time to preparation for contracting, for applications for Trust status and to other issues on the new management agenda.

More mundane changes to routine data collection were also imposing additional work on relevant staff. 1987-88, the first full year of the RM Initiative, was the first year for collecting data according to the guidelines of the Körner Steering Committee (1982-84). Staff at the sites found it necessary to spend time clarifying the Körner definitions, notably that of the consultant episode, and in implementing and operating new data collection systems.

Finally, and by way of background, being part of the high-profile RM Initiative imposed its own costs. Principal among these were the demands on time of the steady stream of visitors wanting to know more about RM. All of the sites organised open days, and most held regular sessions for nurses, medical records staff and others. Staff were regularly invited to talk at conferences and other events. Some of the key figures at the sites estimated that they have spent one-two days per week over long periods on these duties. Together these activities had a substantial opportunity cost to each site, and there is a general feeling that progress would have been faster had the burden been less. The roll out of RM did not help here, since it greatly enlarged the numbers of people wanting to find out about RM.

RM IMPLEMENTATION

Against that complex background estimates were nevertheless obtained from documentation provided by the sites for the costs of RM. More precisely the figures in Box 5.5 represent the cost of the additional resources committed to the RM projects and directly to the RM process. (More detailed figures for the sites are contained in Buxton *et al.*, 1991.)

Taking the total figures shown, the range of additional expenditure in the period was from £354,000 to £2.604 million. The very low figure for Arrowe Park, reflects that its main programme of computer implementation occurred after 1990. The figures for all other sites are well in excess of £1 million, and thus notably higher than the £400-600,000 originally estimated in the original Health Notice.

Even these figures can be argued to under-represent the full investment costs at at least two of the sites, Arrowe Park and Royal Hampshire, where concurrently a HIS was introduced. Whilst it is possible to argue that these operational systems, that provide for example computer ordering and reporting of diagnostic tests directly from, and to, terminals on the wards, are conceptually quite distinct from the management support systems that characterise the computer investment in RM, in practice it is not possible to separate benefits (real or perceived) that accrue from RM and from the HIS. Given also that other sites have comparable elements available within their RM technology - Guy's has a results reporting system, and Pilgrim facilities for one - it may be more meaningful to consider the total costs of RM and HIS. Taking an inclusive perspective, the costs for Arrowe Park and the Royal Hampshire are very much higher. Arrowe Park was in the midst of

Box 5.5 Costs of implementing RM (November 86 - March 90) £ thousand

	Arrowe Park	Freeman	Guy's	Huddersfield	Pilgrim	Royal Hampshire
Staff costs	255	282	1,141	616	385	276
Consultancy	8	377	355	330	35	117
Hardware and software	67	951	1,087	1,143	853	666
Training*	-	-	21	48	32	40
Other	24	41	-	222	27	57
Total	354	1,651	2,604	2,359	1,332	1,156
Ward ordering/ reporting	1,000	-	-	-	-	4,228
Department of Health contribution	280	793	1,038	1,171	485	943

* Provided externally; training using additional internal resources is included under staff costs.

implementing its system, and the investment to the end of 1990-91 was estimated to be around £3.2 million. But even this figure does not include their facilities management contract (over £0.5 million per annum). The estimated total investment in HIS alone was £5 million over 7 years. The Royal Hampshire had completed the implementation of the in-patient elements of their HIS system, and their investment up to the end of 1989-90 was around £5.4 million. Both of these figures must be treated with caution, since work continues at both sites: but they provide a guide to the order of the investments made.

The comparison of costs between sites is further complicated by differences in purchasing arrangements for hardware and software. Four of the sites (Guy's, Freeman, Huddersfield and Pilgrim) purchased hardware and software outright. The range of costs for these sites was from £850,000 to £1.064 million. Arrowe Park was purchasing its RM database during 1990-91: including the estimate for this year, the total cost of hardware and software would be £977,000. The Royal Hampshire has a facilities management contract: excluding that contract the figure is £640,000, including it for five years, the figure is approximately £1.207 million (at 1989-90 prices). This latter figure does, though, include some maintenance and support costs not included in the figures quoted for the other sites.

Estimates of the value of existing resources - principally staff - devoted to the implementation of RM have been particularly difficult to determine. They include the time of both district and unit staff, whose involvement has varied during the course of implementation. However, estimates provided by some of the sites suggest that they have ranged in value from 20 per cent to 45 per cent of the additional investment costs.

The costs discussed above do not reflect all the important inputs to the projects: in particular, sites have in some cases received 'free' consultancy time or 'preferred' deals with suppliers, as part of the companies' own commercial needs to develop products for RM. Additionally, individuals within the hospitals have been involved on an informal basis, perhaps so that they can advise on some aspect of implementation, or lend their authority to effect some desired change; and on a more formal basis, as in the prototyping of a computer system. The time costs to these individuals have typically been low compared with those more centrally involved.

Since the development of RM was not complete by the end of the evaluation, sites were asked to estimate the total final financial costs of implementation. This proved impossible in practice, since RM is increasingly linked to post-Review developments. The best indication of future costs was the bids made for further developmental funding for 1990-91 (Box 5.6). These bids emphasise that the investment in RM was by no means complete at some of the sites.

Box 5.6   Bids for additional funding for 1990-91

	Total (£ thousands)	Out-patients (£ thousands)	Department of Health contribution (£ thousands)
Arrowe Park (1) (with Clatterbridge)	1,103	N/A	1,081
Freeman	184	74	129
Guy's (2)	1,737	4	397
Huddersfield (3)	382	50	N/A
Pilgrim	450	N/A	414
Royal Hampshire	120	N/A	309

These figures include further developments for both in- and out-patients.

(1)   HIS investment, for Arrowe Park alone, estimated at £987,000.

(2)   Funds requested in 1990-91 bid: not expected to commit this sum within the financial year.

(3)   Includes extension of RM to St Luke's Hospital (principally long-stay patients).

It is difficult to put into perspective these estimates of investment and implementation costs, not only because of the difficulties of distinguishing between those committed to the RM projects and to the process, but also because there is no framework for direct comparison. Nonetheless, it is possible to develop a framework based on estimates of the additional costs per unit of output over given time periods. Box 5.7 converts, for each site, the costs from Box 5.5 plus the relevant additional planned expenditure from Box 5.6 into a present value at 1989-90 prices. Actual expenditures are adjusted by the Health Services Price Index and discounted at the Treasury rate of 6 per cent. Then, taking two alternative estimates of the useful life of the 'investment' in RM (of five years and ten years) an annual equivalent charge is calculated - in effect 'the investment cost per year of use'. These figures are then related to the most appropriate available measure of workload of the hospitals, in-patient episodes including day cases. Finally, these costs per in-patient episode are expressed as a percentage of the average cost per in-patient episode.

Inevitably, there must be caveats associated with these estimates: most obviously, future developments will in some cases be across more than one site, (for example the RM database at Freeman will be used by the two other acute hospitals in the district), so that costs are shared; and total costs of developments in areas such as out-patients cannot be predicted. But the figures are based primarily on sums already committed, and are used here as the best available guide to the scale of the investment associated with RM.

In terms of the annual equivalent charge, the figures indicate a wide range of costs. When related to activity measures the costs ranges are still considerable but the absolute magnitude fairly modest: £7.80 to £27.30 per patient episode for an assumed capital life of five years, or an add-on of between 1.4 per cent and 3.3 per cent to patient costs. Similarly, for a capital life of ten years, the costs range from £4.50 to £15.60 per episode, or an add-on to patient costs of 0.8 per cent to 2.4 per cent.

If one includes HIS, the costs for the two sites are £27.60 (Arrowe Park) and £64.30 (Royal Hampshire) per patient episode for an assumed capital life of five years, or an add-on of 4.9 per cent and 11.3 per cent respectively, a much more substantial addition to costs.

RM PROCESSES

Whilst it was not possible to isolate all the resources committed to the on-going process of RM, it was possible to identify key staff at sub-unit level who bore a great deal of the responsibility for running RM. Box 5.8 presents illustrative estimates of

Box 5.7   Combined RM and HIS investment costs

	Arrowe Park (RM)	Arrowe Park (RM + HIS)	Freeman (RM)	Guy's (RM)
Present value of capital and implementation cost (£ millions)	£1.32	£3.19	£1.90	£4.23
Annual equivalent charge (£ thousands):				
- five years	£314	£1,113	£450	£1,004
- ten years	£280		£258	£575
Annual number of in-patient episodes (+ day cases)	40,408	40,408	39,985	36,820
Additional cost per episode:				
- five years	£7.80	£27.60	£11.30	£27.30
- ten years	£4.50	N/A	£6.50	£15.60
Total cost per episode	£566	£566.25	£718	£961
Percentage addition to cost (per cent):				
- five years	1.4	4.9	1.6	2.8
- ten years	0.8	N/A	0.9	1.6

Box 5.7 (continued)

	Huddersfield (RM)	Pilgrim (RM)	Royal Hampshire (RM)	Royal Hampshire (RM + HIS)
Present value of capital and implementation cost (£ millions)	£2.84	£1.77	£1.38	£5.796
Annual equivalent charge (£ thousands):				
- five years	£674	£420	£431	£1,480
- ten years	£386	£240	£305	
Annual number of in-patient episodes (+ day cases)	26,144	26,388	23,012	23,012
Additional cost per episode:				
- five years	£25.80	£15.90	£18.00	£64.30
- ten years	£14.80	£9.10	£12.80	£39.30
Total cost per episode	£897	£728	£541	£540.74
Percentage addition to cost (per cent):				
- five years	2.9	2.2	3.3	11.3
- ten years	1.6	1.3	2.4	6.9

Box 5.8   Sub-unit costs, 1989-90

The costs presented here are estimates of the total annual cost of RM for key staff at sub-unit level. They reflect both new, additional costs of management at this level and the formalisation of pre-existing arrangements into new structures.

Sub-unit 1	*(£ thousands)*
Clinical director	12
Business manager	11
Nurse manager	20
Ward sisters	5
Unit office	6
Total	54

Sub-unit 1 is a surgical sub-unit with a budget of £1.24 million. Estimates are given here based on the time the Clinical Director spends on RM, the full salaries of nurse and business managers; the time spent by ward sisters on RM-related activities, derived from questionnaires; and the contribution of administrative and clerical staff in supporting RM.

Sub-unit 2	*(£ thousands)*
Clinical director	20
Nurse manager (part time)	5
Business manager (part year)	10
Medical records	7
Total	42

Sub-unit 2 is a medical sub-unit with a budget of £1.57 million. Estimates are divided as for sub-unit 1.

Sub-unit 3	*(£ thousands)*
Clinical director	10
Nurse/business manager	22
Ward sisters	4
Administrative and clerical	3
Total	38

Sub-unit 3 is a surgical sub-unit with a budget of £1.45 million. The basis of the estimates is the same as for sub-unit 1, except that the administrative and clerical time includes a secretary specifically 'seconded' from normal duties to help develop a computer system for six months.

the costs of running sub-units using data provided by the sites, and our own judgements of which staff were involved in RM.

But involvement in RM does not end at sub-unit level. Evidence for the time spent on RM-related activities by consultants and ward sisters is available from the questionnaires and interviews. Consultants were asked how much time they actually spent and how much time they felt it was appropriate for them to spend on RM-related work. The values for actual and appropriate time were broadly similar and are summarised in Box 5.9.

Box 5.9 Time commitment per consultant

- audit meetings per month: up to one session;
- directorate meetings per month: 0-2 hours;
- coding per month: 0-2 hours;
- review of their own work per month: up to one session;
- training or being trained for RM: negligible.

Ward sisters across the sites spent relatively small amounts of time on RM-related activities, such as audit and directorate business meetings and reviewing the work of their wards; certainly, less than consultants. Above ward level the involvement of senior nurses and directors of nursing services in RM-related processes is difficult to comment upon. It could be argued that sub-unit nurse managers must have been devoting all their time to RM simply by virtue of their position.

It is clear that in some sites structures were still evolving, and it is reasonable to suppose that the senior nurses there were still taking on tasks, recognisable as RM, which they did not perform before. These include the active management of nursing budgets.

The amount of training provided by, and to, nurses varied hugely both in organisation and quantity between the sites. The Royal Hampshire necessarily provided an extensive support system through the project nurses to introduce HIS on to each ward. Other sites relied on training and support from project nurses when computer systems were introduced.

Ward sisters in general reported that they had provided or received little training in the previous twelve months, ranging from none to three hours. A few nurses did, however, report that they had spent two-three days being trained; and a few also that they had provided several days' training to other nurses. This was focused on computer systems rather than on RM generally.

The question arises of the opportunity costs of time spent by staff away from their patients. Evidence from interviews and observation of meetings suggests that some of the people most closely involved, notably clinical directors, had simply worked longer hours, so that the costs fell on themselves rather than on patients (Brooks, 1990). Many consultants and nurses had thought about the trade-off and came to the conclusion that even where it involved time away from patients, it had been worth making.

The burden of both implementing and running RM fell particularly heavily on a small core of individuals at the sites. Project managers reported that they had regularly put in very long days over the whole period of the project. Similarly, some consultants committed to RM had made considerable time investments; one such example is given in Box 5.10. This is representative of those whose enthusiasm and drive lead them to become involved in all aspects of RM, and not of the wider body of consultants, nurses and managers.

There were significant changes in the way that some activities were carried out. One example here was clinical coding. At all sites prior to RM, coding was a centralised medical records function - as it still is at Guy's - and was divorced from service provision. At the five other sites this arrangement changed and coding staff were attached to particular specialties. Coding became seen as a joint venture with junior medical staff and consultants, but generally this change increased the cost of coding.

Direct cost savings and benefit realisation

Finally, there is the issue of direct cost savings resulting from RM. It is reasonable to expect that RM (and particularly its information technology aspects) would in part replace tasks and activities previously undertaken, so rendering them unnecessary or speeding them up. This automation effect should be seen as quite distinct from the effects the information and management systems can subsequently have on the organisation - in informing, indeed perhaps transforming, the pattern of (health) services provided and the way that services are produced and delivered (Ernst and Young, 1990). The automation effect should lead to reductions in the resource inputs required for those existing tasks, so potentially providing an element of cost saving to set against the running costs of the new technology. Any savings or benefits achieved of this sort are then conceptually quite distinct from savings or benefits that may result from using the data, or from management systems.

Box 5.10   On being a 'lead consultant'

Many people at the sites have made a major personal commitment to RM. Outlined here is the time spent by one consultant who was a member of a hospital's project team during the three months April-June 1989.

The time spent on RM each week averaged some 10.5 hours. This included:

> directorate meetings
> other meetings, including RM project team
> management board related activities
> directorate-related activities
> development of computer systems.

The time excludes all audit, but includes both developments and on-going processes associated with RM. The activities included review of routine reports and preparation for meetings.

In late-1989, the consultant reported that the time commitment had been greater than he had anticipated, and was alarmed at the slow rate of development of the new information systems, which meant that the whole project would take longer than anyone had imagined. By mid-1990, however, things were looking brighter, and the consultant felt that they were finally making real progress. 'Finally, I can see how it will all work properly.'

It is on such 'first-order' resource savings that the so called 'benefit-realisation' programmes have tended to focus, encouraged by the claims of the systems suppliers. Formalised assessment of potential savings was carried out for Royal Hampshire and for Wirral, in each case relating particularly to the HIS. The initial aim at the Royal Hampshire was to make sufficient cash-releasing changes to pay, in the first year of operation (1989-90), for the running costs of the system at the hospital, and early documentation suggested an eventual saving of 4-8 per cent of nursing time. In the event at the Royal Hampshire slightly more than 4 per cent of the nursing budget was withdrawn to contribute to the running costs of the system. A similar expectation was reported in the Wirral plans to convert some of the organisational benefits accruing from the system into financial savings, which would offset the operational costs of the system from 1992-93 onwards (Wirral General Hospital, Outline Application for Trust Status).

A detailed ex-ante appraisal of the expected costs and benefits of a hospital information system was undertaken for Wirral Health Authority in 1987-88, and this indicated a district wide benefit realisation of £1 million per annum, representing 37 per cent of the total quantifiable benefits compared to an expected running cost of £0.75 million (DHSS, 1988). Of this £1 million, £0.58 million was estimated to come from nursing, and £0.21 million from medical records and administration staffing. This expectation seems to echo the much earlier analysis of the first implementation of a hospital information system in the early 1970s at El Camino Hospital, California (Coffey, 1980). This had found that the system appeared to have reduced nursing costs per patient by 5 per cent, it may have increased *overall* hospital costs by up to 3.9 per cent (although this increase was not statistically significant).

Such studies emphasise the importance of distinguishing between the direct resource implications of new technology and the managerial decisions about the resources to be allocated to particular tasks.

CONCLUSION

It has been difficult to separate out the costs associated with RM, both conceptually and practically. It has, however, been possible to distinguish the additional investment costs in RM, which range from £354,000 to £2.604 million. This range increased from £1.354 million to £5.384 million if the costs of the concurrent investment in HIS are included. Relating the costs of RM to the costs of the hospitals as a whole gives a clearer indication of the cost impact. Considering RM as an investment over five years the additional cost per patient episode ranges from 1.4 per cent to 3.3 per cent (or 4.9 per cent to 11.3 per cent including the HIS at Arrowe Park and Royal Hampshire). These costs, however, exclude the cost of the time of existing staff involved in implementing the project and running the RM process. Estimates from particular sites suggest that such costs may add a further 20-45 per cent. What is impossible to isolate at this stage is what will be the net costs of running a fully developed RM system, when such a state is eventually reached.

Chapter 6

BENEFITS OF RM

INTRODUCTION

For some people, the success of RM rests or falls on the change in process it engenders. If, as a unit manager, you perceive the problem to be one of an absence, in the 'traditional' hospital management process, of a mechanism to get clinicians to take responsibility for the effects of their activity on budgets, then a successful process change to RM may be an end in itself. Or if, as a senior clinician, you perceive the problem to be a lack of control over the balance of resources available for use in your specialty, then again a successful change in process to clinical directorates with management responsibility for budgets may be a sufficient indication of success. And to the extent that RM was about achieving medical and nursing 'ownership' of the system, of establishing accurate patient activity data, and introducing patient case mix planning and costing, then process changes are indeed measures of success.

Certainly much of the effort at the six pilot sites has been initially focused on implementing a coherent management process. Chapter 4 has described fully the process changes, and whilst achievement to date is variable, there is no doubt that significant improvement in the management processes has occurred at most of the sites. This might therefore be viewed as an important indicator of the success of the RM Initiative, *providing* the evidence suggests that the RM process can *potentially* provide a means to a better service.

The inherent logic of the conceptual model of Box 4.1 is that, for example, through the RM process collaboration between members of different professional groups takes place. They bring together and pool relevant knowledge, arrive at agreed decisions about a course of action, have authority (and resources) to act on that decision and go ahead to change and improve the service they deliver. Our study has shown that the simple conceptual model can be translated into practice, most strikingly at the sub-unit level. Clinicians, nurses and business managers can discuss and change the allocation of resources, and use improved information available to them to more closely monitor the situation. It is thus quite reasonable to suppose that the delivery of services might be improved as a result of these new ways of working. Process change is therefore an indicator of potential success.

But Chapters 3 and 4 have indicated that there are a number of factors which influence whether or not the RM process actually leads to improvements in services. These include: the extent to which RM has 'taken hold' at a site; the availability of reliable data on which to base decisions; the ability of participants to identify desired benefits and work out how to realise them; and, the availability of the appropriate resources, including staff with the necessary skills. It is therefore not sufficient that process change has taken place; the change in process needs to be put to good effect. Process is a necessary but not a sufficient condition. The principal objective, as clearly set down in the Annex to HN(86)34 was to achieve measurable improvements in patient care, and the requirement for such evidence was reiterated in the October 1989 Interim Evaluation by the CCSC (1989).

This Chapter reviews the available data on outcome benefits in terms of seven main elements of evidence. The first of these draws on the available routine quantitative data (presented in Appendix 2) on the *overall changes in performance* of the six sites. The subsequent three sections draw on our detailed research material from interviews, documents, meetings, etc., and focus on specific examples of benefits, in terms of three types of outcomes - *service production benefits*, *service activity benefits* and *patient outcome benefits*. The final three sections are concerned more with overall *perceptions* of benefit of key groups at the sites. These elements draw principally on evidence from the questionnaires to *consultants* and to *nurses*, and our many interviews and meetings with *key managers* (particularly UGMs) at the six sites. The chapter then concludes with a discussion of what these various partial elements imply for an overall assessment of the extent and timing of the benefits from RM.

THE OVERALL PERFORMANCE OF THE SIX SITES

Available quantitative data on the performance of each of the six sites over the period of the RM Initiative, can be compared with the data for all acute hospitals in the NHS as a generic control. This quantitative data is important at two levels. The first is that *potentially*, it might show a clear and consistent picture in its own terms. An improving performance at each site, and collectively a performance for the six that was clearly superior to that of the NHS more generally, would represent strong supporting evidence of the beneficial effect of RM. This performance might show improved efficiency in terms of output activity per unit of input. The second level is that it serves as a background to the more detailed observations about the sites, and helps to put the circumstances of the units into context.

The available data is presented in Appendix 2. As the introduction to that Appendix explains in more detail, there were considerable problems in obtaining data. For routine data that should be available for all units, the introduction of the Körner data requirements from 1987-88 onwards produced a major discontinuity with earlier data series. Thus broadly comparable data is only available for three years -

1987-88, 1988-89 and 1989-90. Moreover, it has resulted in data for the first two years being recognised by most in the NHS as particularly unreliable. This restriction means the lack of a real pre-RM Initiative baseline and of data for 1990-91, when most of the sites might be seen as having had a nearly complete RM process in place.

It is impossible to draw clear unambiguous conclusions from this data. The national data for the acute sector shows the discontinuities in definitions, and, possibly as a result, rather strange movement in key indicators. It appears that in-patient, out-patient and accident and emergency activity levels fell in 1988-89 but rose again in 1989-90, as did length of stay (though this latter figure is for a limited range of specialties). Day case activity has risen steadily. Cost data nationally is extremely limited.

The performance of the sites, in these simplistic terms, is not consistent:

- At Arrowe Park in-patient activity rose slightly in each year; out-patient activity followed the national pattern of a decline in the middle year, as did accident and emergency. Day case activity however fell. Length of stay declined steadily but in-patient and out-patient unit costs rose. The budgetary context has been one of a slight decline in real terms in 1989-90.

- Freeman Hospital data showed steadily increasing, day case and accident and emergency activity. Out-patient activity increased in 1988-89 but declined slightly in 1989-90. Length of stay at Freeman steadily fell, as did in-patient costs, but out-patient costs have risen over the period. The budgetary context was one of a significant increase in 1988-89 and a small fall in 1989-90.

- At Guy's the picture is more complex still. In-patient activity rose in 1988-89 and fell in 1989-90; day case activity increased steadily; accident and emergency declined steadily. Length of stay increased steadily. In-patient costs increased in 1988-89 but fell slightly in 1989-90: out-patient costs rose dramatically and then fell even more dramatically. At Guy's the hospital budget increased in 1988-89 and then fell again in 1989-90.

- In Huddersfield, in-patient activity declined slightly in 1988-89 and then rose in 1989-90. Out-patient, accident and emergency and day cases increased each year. Length of stay fell steadily. In-patient costs rose considerably in 1988-89 but returned to their previous level in 1989-90. Out-patient costs, however, fell significantly in 1988-89. Again the picture was of a budget increase in 1988-89 and a fall again in 1989-90.

- For Pilgrim in-patient activity and day case activity rose in 1988-89 and then fell in 1989-90. Out-patients and accident and emergency rose steadily. Length of stay fell in each year. In-patient costs per episode fell in 1988-89 but rose in 1989-90; out-patient costs increased considerably. Pilgrim enjoyed a small increase in budget each year.

■ For the Royal Hampshire in-patient activity levels appear to have increased; out-patient activity fell then increased; day case activity rose significantly then fell slightly; and accident and emergency fell steadily. Length of stay data is not available. In-patient costs rose in 1988-89 and fell in 1989-90 whilst out-patient costs did the reverse. The Royal Hampshire also enjoyed an increase in budget each year.

The overall impression is that the sites may have out-performed the national data in this three year period on such key indicators as length of stay. But no clear picture emerges, and many of the changes could well be quirks of the data rather than reflections of reality. Even were the data totally accurate, the performance of the sites would anyway need to be judged in relationship to local circumstances: for example to local financial constraints or to planned changes in local patterns of service. And to do this would require consideration of a longer time series of reliable, consistent data. The figures as presently available merely emphasise how difficult it is currently to make meaningful comparisons of performance between units.

SERVICE PRODUCTION BENEFITS

By service production benefits we mean *improvements* in the way in which resources are used to produce output: for example, the allocation of resources between specialties; the organisation of patient services; patterns of patient management; use of support facilities/departments.

A number of examples of *changes* in service production can be given, in each case apparently the result of the RM process. These range from small changes instituted by individual clinicians, to policy changes or changes of priority at sub-unit level, to major shifts between specialties in resources available at unit level.

Some changes reflect the use of delegated budgetary responsibility and flexibility to sub-units or clinical groups to agree to use resources to improve the environment and organisational arrangements for patients. For example, funds were used to provide a grieving room, a paediatric department decided to appoint an out-patient receptionist, so reducing the number of complaints about out-patient clinics. At one site a staff grade nephrologist was employed with money saved on dialysis fluids. The admission of waiting list patients was rescheduled to avoid bringing in patients on a Sunday, so reducing the numbers of staff on duty at expensive un-social hours.

Additionally there were several instances of active consideration of moving to five-day wards.

Nurses pointed to the better organisation of ward routines and more flexible rostering. With better data and a more questioning approach, nurse staffing had been more appropriately matched to needs on the ward at particular times of the day. This had allowed a later start to the 'patient day'. The artificial timing of the end of the afternoon shift, which does not coincide with any particular aspect of clinical activity on the patients day, had been scrapped. With a greater control over the way the budget is spent, ward sisters have changed their skill mix to reflect their development of nursing practice into team or primary nursing. At one site three wards piloting this flexible approach reduced sickness/absence rates from an average of 8.5 per cent to 2.5 per cent.

> I am now more aware of the financial requirements within my ward. Also there is more information to the other ward staff. Quality of care delivered and work carried out is now more in question, which makes staff more responsible.
>
> Ward Sister

One site used the RM data to review carefully whether or not an additional anaesthetist was required. It was decided that by appropriate rescheduling of anaesthetists' theatre sessions and their ITU sessions, an additional anaesthetist would not be needed. Similarly, review of activity had made consultants realise that some facilities were being underutilised, and this had led to reallocation of services between wards.

At many of the sites RM led to, or at least coincided with and facilitated, the introduction of agreed clinical management policies for specific groups of patients. Standardised policies for management of common conditions (including myocardial infarction, haematuresis, stone removal, acute chest pain and thromboembolism prophylaxis) were cited as examples, reflecting a fairly general view that sub-unit organisational arrangements made it easier for clinicians to work together, rather than as individuals. These cases appear to rest on the organisational changes, rather than on the availability of detailed individual patient data. By contrast, incidences were still cited where improved data clearly identified that resources such as theatre lists or clinic sessions allocated to individual clinicians were underutilised, but no mechanism existed to make those concerned release these resources.

Not all changes in service production were clear improvements. Public attention was drawn to the decision at Guy's to cut out-patient prescribing to reduce costs by £59,000 a year (*The Independent*, 11 August 1990). Some respondents from Guy's viewed that decision critically, as an undesirable outcome of the RM process. This illustrates two points of importance: (i) the extent to which RM is the cause of a problem or the vehicle for finding a solution, and (ii) the extent to which it is possible to compare outcomes with what would have happened in the absence of RM. The publicly stated position was that this action at Guy's was better than closing beds.

> RM has meant care over prescribing more expensive drugs. Much less out-patient prescribing.
>
> Consultant

SERVICE ACTIVITY BENEFITS

Service activity benefits are defined here as concerning the quantity and mix of patient services delivered - numbers of in-patients, out-patients, day cases, etc.; length of stay; waiting times, readmission or reattendance rates. Without fully reliable data on the total case mix of the sites over a period of time, it is difficult to take a firm view of their overall position. Here again the main evidence is of illustrative examples and, again, such examples vary considerably.

Some clinicians believed that improved information had led to changes in clinical management which had reduced lengths of stay and increased patient throughput. For example, review of patient data led to reduced lengths of stay and greater throughput within obstetrics and gynaecology. This had released beds for other departments (though these had not yet been reassigned).

More generally, we observed the way in which the structure of a clinical directorate provided the framework for agreed planning of service restrictions. Box 6.1 provides an example of this conscious planning of activity against available budget, even if the available data was still imperfect. At a unit level the clinically focused management board and sub-units *appeared* to help one of the sites to handle the cut-back in service activity necessary to meet a financial crisis. This represents an interesting case-study summarised in Box 6.2. Similar claims were of course presented as key evidence in the early success of the Guy's structure of management board and directorates. There too those involved in introducing the new structure in 1985 were convinced that it had been essential in enabling the hospital to meet

Box 6.1 Special meeting to discuss sub-unit over-expenditure

Present: clinical director, three other consultants, nurse manager, business manager, researcher.

The clinical director opened. They were in month six of the financial year. The projected unit overspend for the year was £500,000. The directorate's current position £60,000 over budget according to their statement: but this figure could well be wrong. The nurse staffing figures for one ward were definitely overstated; the drug budget figures were difficult to interpret; and the medical and surgical supplies expenditure had mysteriously risen twelve-fold earlier in the year. The business manager had been striving to get better data from the finance department, but had met with little success. The business manager reported that the finance people were grappling with a new system of charging to sub-units, and were still unclear how to do it so as to provide stable costings.

The clinical director said there were two broad strategies. One was to accept the £60,000 figure and 'go for broke', close the hospital to all but emergency cases for a period. This raised ethical problems. The other was to state that the service could not be cut, and any overspend would have to be carried forward. Consultant 1 said they really had to have reliable data before making any decision: perhaps they should spend money on outside help to generate it. Consultant 2 agreed: but felt they really couldn't cut their service any further. The nurse manager pointed to particular problems caused by Project 2000: they could not attract enough care assistants (who had recently replaced student nurses), and had instead to employ agency nurses. Consultant 2 wondered whether any cuts made now wouldn't turn out to be permanent. Anyway, what was wrong with an overdraft? The clinical director said there was a Department of Health directive that units not be overspent by April 1991. Consultant 1 wondered if this was inviolate. Consultant 3 was reminded of CEPOD, which had come out against out of hours emergency work, yet as they closed wards and reduced theatre sessions there would be more of it. Surely they had to resist short term pressures, and look to the long term: they could not cut their service without then failing to fulfil their obligations to the local population. Anyway, they couldn't close any more beds since they were already at the minimum for the emergency service. They were now trading-off savings and efficiency: making the former would reduce the latter. The clinical director said that he had asked for a number of options to be costed, but felt they would have to 'close' if the £60,000 figure turned out to be accurate. The other consultants agreed, reluctantly, that this might be necessary. The director would do three things: look into the possibility of carrying over the overspend; advocate help to get better financial data; and if it proved necessary, decide to close their wards to elective patients for a period.

Box 6.2   RM and a financial crisis

At one of the sites a significant financial crisis, a major overspend
projected to be £1.2 million (equivalent to 6 per cent of total annual
budget) emerged at the end of the summer. Both unit and district agreed
that the problem largely came about due to factors external to the unit,
principally the level of excess cost inflation and the effects of nurse
regrading. Although early warning of the problem was delayed because of
the information system changes - a new system of monthly reporting on
activity/expenditure was not fully operational but the old was already in
abeyance - the impressive feature was the collective ownership of the
problem by the board, their 'amazing' commitment to right the situation,
and their level of agreement on a non-arbitrary pattern of 'cuts', which was
then complemented by the ability of the directorates to deliver the
necessary reductions in activity. (Nevertheless the unit ended up overspent
by £650,000 or 3 per cent of its budget.)

the enormous (largely RAWP-based) cuts in budget (Smith and Chantler, 1987; Chantler, 1989).

However in the case cited in Box 6.2, recognising the undoubted benefit of the ability of the management organisation to handle such a financial situation in a positive way, does not remove the concern that the information systems, particularly financial, may have exacerbated the initial problem. Certainly it has been a recurrent observation that the supply of information has often deteriorated before it has improved, as old and imperfect but functioning systems have been abandoned ahead of the ability of the new systems to deliver improved data.

PATIENT OUTCOMES

At this point the tenuous chain of linkage between the RM process and even illustrative examples of benefit stretched to breaking. We simply cannot point at this stage to changes, good or bad, in patient outcomes - in quality of life or survival - that can be associated with RM. Many of the exemplar changes referred to in the previous two sections clearly aim to improve outcomes, but as yet the data systems do not routinely permit the monitoring of the impact of such changes on patient outcomes.

It is important to stress that the routine systems still include virtually no patient outcome data, despite the repeated desire from clinicians to link inputs to outcomes. At Huddersfield, outcome data is not routinely included across the hospital but is included as a special study for geriatric patients. Analysis of post-discharge outcome measures used by geriatricians has lead to a shift of resources to provide improved home-care support to avoid the observed deterioration in patient-dependency post-discharge.

At Freeman, a research study has been undertaken collaboratively with Clinical Accountability, Service Planning and Evaluation (CASPE) of the King's Fund. The aim of this work is to establish whether and how appropriate information on patient outcomes can be collected on a routine basis and used alongside existing RM data in the management of health care. Work is going on relating to out-patient care of diabetic patients, cholecystectomy, rheumatology, arthroplasty, geriatric care and coronary disease. These exceptions serve to highlight the general situation that outcomes are not yet a routine part of RM data collection, and that if they are to become so special exercises will be required.

Whilst not strictly a measure of outcome, waiting times for out-patient visits are a very visible indicator to patients of the quality of process. One clinician monitored indicated that as a result of the fact that the RM data showed that he saw newly referred patients more quickly than his colleagues, he had levelled his practice down to that of his colleagues. Without appropriate incentives, responses to information may not be as desired!

PERCEPTIONS OF CONSULTANTS AND NURSES

The perceptions of consultants and nurses, the main service providers, are an important barometer of the whole RM exercise. More clearly than any outside observer could hope to see, they have a sense of what is going on and changing in the hospitals. Like the outside observer, they may have some difficulty in defining this development called RM, and of correctly linking this as a cause to the effects they observe. But in that one of the key aims of the initiative has been to involve doctors and nurses in management, then their perceptions of the overall value of the process are crucial to its success (see Appendix 1).

> It is hard to say how much these changes have been brought about by resource management, but they seem to occur more quickly.
>
> > Consultant, referring to various restrictions
> > in availability of resources.

Based on a survey of the views of consultants in the directorates (or their equivalents) of general medicine and general surgery at each of the six sites, Box 6.3 summarises consultants perceptions. They were positive about the effect of RM on encouraging good working practices, and remained positive that RM *would* eventually improve the care of their patients. But they tended to disagree that it was already improving care, or that it helped them to provide care at lower cost.

In essence, it confirms our other evidence that the process had improved but as yet there was little evidence of improvement in outcome. Overall, they nevertheless viewed RM somewhat more positively than when they had first become involved in the experiment.

What is clear from the specific comments in the questionnaires was that many respondents perceived RM as having helped in a context of falling or inadequate resources, but this did not lead them to a positive view of it having assisted them to improve care. (It is a matter of very relevant speculation, but speculation nevertheless, as to whether in the future context of contracts, consultants will see RM more positively as giving them the basis to attract funds by offering greater efficiency or higher quality.)

Box 6.3   Consultants' perceptions

	Strongly agree	Agree	No opinion	Disagree	Strongly disagree
I think that RM encourages good working practice	9	41	16	8	0
I think that RM *is* improving the care of my patients	3	13	20	33	4
I think that RM *will* improve the care of my patients	4	33	19	19	0
I think RM helps me to provide care at lower cost	4	21	17	28	4

	More positive		No change		Less positive
Do you feel more or less positive about the value of RM than when you first became involved?	25		33		17

It has enabled resource shortfalls to be dealt with in a more rational manner.

Contraction of services are a result of team discussions.

With falling resources, RM has become a method of effectively administering cuts rather than maximising benefits.

Consultants

The views of nurses (see Box 6.4) were remarkably similar to those of the consultants. They, too, tended to agree that RM encouraged good working practices, and that it *would* improve patient care. But they were divided as to whether it was currently improving care or helping to provide care at lower cost. Nevertheless, overall the majority were more positive about RM than when they first had become involved.

The nursing sisters in their written comments frequently indicated that RM had made them more aware of costs and of budgetary constraints, but several worried that the information systems were time-consuming and reduced their time with patients. They were hopeful that RM could lead to improvements in care, but saw little current evidence. A few feared that it would lead to tighter and tighter control on resources and declining standards.

I feel more aware of cost related to patient care. Our clinical director seems more aware of our problems.

It makes everyone more aware of the need for cost effective care - as long as standards are maintained.

It appears to have little positive benefit towards areas and involves a lot of extra work. It will not be successful until we obtain the sort of information we need from it.

Ward Sisters

Whilst there is nothing close to unanimity of individual views, both consultants and nurses as a group across the sites seem to subscribe to an agreement with the ideas of RM, to there being an extant improvement in process and to continued hopes for improvements in care in the future.

Box 6.4   Nurses' perceptions

	Strongly agree	Agree	No opinion	Disagree	Strongly disagree
I think that RM encourages good working practice	4	21	3	5	0
I think that RM *is* improving the care of my patients	1	13	8	10	2
I think that RM *will* improve the care of my patients	2	24	4	4	0
I think RM helps me to provide care at lower cost	0	11	10	11	0

	More positive		No change		Less positive
Do you feel more or less positive about the value of RM than when you first became involved?	21		8		5

PERCEPTIONS OF KEY MANAGERS

Over the course of the study we regularly took soundings of the overall opinions of RM from the key managers involved locally (particularly the UGMs) through one-to-one interviews. Their opinions ranged from fairly to very positive, although all expressed some element of frustration over delays or problems, particularly in instituting the computer system developments and in getting reliable data.

They all welcomed and emphasised the cultural change that had taken place. Commitment, collaboration, involvement and unity of purpose, were the sort of positive characteristics that had been engendered. Doctors were now involved directly in management, and managers were able to routinely discuss issues of management with them against a better, if not yet perfect, background of activity data. Managers at all sites that had formal sub-unit structures saw these as a key element in RM.

Unit managers saw RM as having significantly helped the units to manage change. Those that had experienced financial problems felt they would have been in a more difficult situation without the new structures. It had helped them deal with long-standing issues that had been discussed for years but it had not been possible to act on, as well as putting the units in a strong position for newer challenges such as contracting.

There appeared to be a managerial view that at most sites the key features of RM were now robust elements of normal life, and RM was 'taken for granted'. But the cultural change was not yet complete and in the last few months RM had ceased to occupy centre-stage. UGMs differed in their views, however, as to whether the NHS reforms had acted as a distraction from RM, as an added reason for it or whether the debate had substantively moved beyond RM to new issues.

Managers expressed a number of on-going concerns. Whilst RM might have continued for longer as an experiment, new information systems took time to implement and it was inevitable that benefits relying on the availability of data would only emerge slowly. There was also a fear expressed, echoing that of the consultants, that resource constraint might eventually ruin RM: experience to date suggests that consultants would accept ownership of budgets and co-operate to control them, but if restrictions continued year in and year out, they might lose heart and lose interest in participating in management. The overriding view of the managers, however, was that none would wish to go back to more traditional ways of managing, and all, given a second chance, would again opt to embark on the implementation of RM.

CONCLUSION

The overall picture concerning benefits of RM is still far from definitive. In terms of specific benefits to patient care there are now a number of good examples of positive changes in delivery of care. We found illustrative examples of service production and service activity changes. But there is a problem in determining causation. Many of the changes cited could have been achieved in other ways, without RM. We have tried to give as examples only those that seem directly linked to the RM process, but proponents of RM may give it credit for other less clearly related changes and critics may point to the fact that similar examples of change could be found in sites without RM. But it is not yet possible to form a general picture of the real magnitudes of such changes, and as yet there is no evidence of effects on patient outcomes.

The data on the overall performance of the sites showed, as one would expect, variable performance in varying circumstances. To the extent that limited comparison could be made with national data the suggestion is probably of better than average performance, taking the six sites together. But the data is unreliable and limited. Analysis of case mix adjusted costs and lengths of stay would allow firmer conclusions but this is not currently feasible.

Nevertheless, the perceptions of staff involved are generally positive - those of key managers very much so. In part, these views reflect the major improvements in management associated with the RM process - improvements that were described in detail in Chapter 4. These changes are seen as beneficial in their own right by those involved. In part, the positive perceptions reflect a continued expectation that RM can increasingly deliver patient care benefits.

Chapter 7

CONCLUSIONS AND IMPLICATIONS

RM AND ITS EVALUATION

RM is a continuous process by which service providers and general managers together determine the strategic and operational commitment of the available resources, doing so in the light of their knowledge of the requirements of, and implications for, the activities involved in delivering patient treatment and care.

This definition incorporates a number of crucial and complex elements which together represent a major change in respect of traditional management practice in the NHS. Service providers are required to involve themselves in both the present and future management of resources. General managers are required to manage resources *with* rather than *for* the service providers. The use of resources becomes formalised in an on-going process that can relate current execution to future plans. And, information systems are available that can accurately record service activities and the resources they consume.

When the RM Initiative was announced in November 1986, it was expected that the six sites would implement a radically new process of management in two years, so permitting a first evaluation to be undertaken in 1988. Four years after the announcement, it was clear that the sites had not completely implemented RM, and equally clear that the scale and complexity of RM was initially underestimated. Increasingly, the recognition has grown that RM involves a fundamental change in the culture of a hospital. The experience of some of those involved in these changes is nicely illustrated in the following quotation.

> There was a touch of heroics about it, a kind of Dunkirk grim-gayness, but also an emerging new feeling of a genuine clinical ownership of the hospital's decision-making and direction-finding. Clinicians were setting priorities and lay managers and administrators lending their efforts to achieve these. We at least began to be able to show in a reasonably quantitative way what we were doing and in grossed-up terms how much it cost to do, where the shortfalls lay, and what was needed to meet them.
>
> H. Keen, 1990

This book is not able to provide a final evaluation of RM at the six pilot sites: in the event, it is simply too early to make such a judgement. It has, however, provided a comprehensive study of the process of implementation, of the nature of RM, of the resources used, and of the benefits to date. The focus has been on the RM Initiative as a whole rather than on a comparison between sites, although specific differences between sites are used to highlight some of the key variables in RM.

This final chapter has three main sections. It commences with a summary of the main conclusions (chapter by chapter) from the evaluation. The second part of the chapter draws out the major lessons that have emerged from the evaluation of the RM Initiative and which are relevant to three different potential audiences. The achievements of the experiment carry important messages for: first, those working in health services who are grappling, or thinking of grappling, with RM in their own sites; second, those concerned with implementing or studying national policy initiatives; and, third, those who are interested or involved in the methodology of evaluating social institutions. Finally, the chapter closes with an overview of the balance of the evidence regarding the overall results of the experiment; first, in respect of hospital management and, second, regarding the wider policy-related elements of RM that were discussed in Chapter 1.

MAJOR CONCLUSIONS

A. Effects of context (see Chapter 1, RM in Context)

■ *RM is sensitive to the environment in which it operates.* Over the course of the experiment this environment changed both nationally, most notably with the NHS Review, and locally. RM reflected these changes.

■ *The NHS Review changed the status of RM.* With the publication of the Review, RM ceased being the subject of an experiment and became national policy. But at the same time the Review imposed other demands. As a result the pilot sites ceased to focus as strongly on RM and progress on the initiative was slowed by the redeployment or loss of key individuals. At some sites the Review led to a polarisation of opinion about RM and the future direction of the unit. The Review has tended to dominate the management agenda at all sites. It has diverted attention from the implementation of RM but also underlined its importance and emphasised its potential contribution in a changed environment.

■ *Participation in a national experiment itself incurred costs.* The sites were the focus of considerable attention from the media, government and various parts of the NHS throughout the experiment. They had to spend a great deal of time in dealing with enquiries and disseminating information, on top of their own efforts to implement RM.

B. Approaches to implementation (see Chapter 2, Project Planning and Management)

■ *Project planning for RM was initially inadequate but improved during implementation.* RM was a major development and required detailed thought and planning, together with a continuous review of objectives and approaches. The scope and quality of planning increased over time but in general project planning was weakened by the absence of clearly articulated information strategies and the difficulties of co-ordinating sub-projects.

■ *Most project managers lacked the necessary authority.* Although there were clearly identified project managers, they generally lacked the authority and the support required to fully effect the changes they were expected to implement. In spite of this, it was impressive how, drawn from different backgrounds and with different expertise and approaches to their work, they were able to effect and influence a range of developments.

C. Progress with implementation (see Chapter 3, The Implementation of RM)

■ *RM represented enormous change.* This was so in respect of the cultural change required from both managers and service providers and also in respect of the major investment made in infrastructure, particularly for computer technology.

■ *Computer systems are incomplete.* The RM databases at most sites are still under development. The focus has been almost exclusively on in-patients - on activity data, and on resources they use. Case mix costing where it exists is still fairly crude. Work is beginning at most of the sites on out-patients. Work on outcome measurement is very patchy, and still mainly at a research stage.

■ *Research and Development was both continuous and incremental.* Throughout the experiment, the sites were the focus of a variety of R and D activities, ranging from patient classification systems to decentralised management.

■ *Quality of data produced improved over time.* The quality of activity data got better as the experiment proceeded, reflecting the commitment of consultants to involvement in the coding process. Progress has, however, been uneven between the sites.

■ *RM for nursing has been implemented separately from the main RM strategies.* The nursing sub-projects were in general managed independently of the main RM projects, although in some instances they received support from project managers and teams. Nursing issues have tended to be somewhat marginalised in the implementation of RM.

■ *Training was insufficient.* All the sites have long been aware that in many respects the training they were able to provide was insufficient. In general they were unable to significantly improve this situation as the experiment proceeded.

■ *The scale of organisation development required for RM was initially underestimated.* It was recognised from the outset that if RM was to be successful, it involved a major cultural change. The full implications of this in terms of helping individuals to understand and adapt were not initially appreciated and provided for, or met by a comprehensive strategy. But sites tried subsequently to respond to the shortfall.

■ *There was a clear move towards sub-unit organisational structures.* By the end of the study five of the six sites had a hospital-wide structure of sub-units, based on clinical specialties. General satisfaction with these new management arrangements was tempered by concern at the lack of support available to the service providers.

D. The nature of RM (see Chapter 4, The RM Process)

■ *RM is a continuous management process.* It consists of five inter-related steps. Service providers determine objectives and priorities for their work. Available resources are allocated accordingly and service providers then exercise responsibility for their management. The resultant resource use and service provision are then monitored and the value of the service provided is reviewed. This review then feeds into the determination of objectives and priorities, and the cycle continues.

■ *The RM process requires the service providers to be actively involved in the management of resources.* This was set as a pre-requisite for the sites wishing to participate in the experiment, although in practice commitment and opportunity varied. Ideally the service providers need to engage with RM at all levels: the individual work set; the sub-unit or specialty; and, the unit. The existence of sub-unit organisational arrangements appears important in formalising and stimulating the service providers' involvement with management.

■ *RM becomes an integral part of general management.* RM represents an enormous change in the way in which hospitals are managed but when it has finally been implemented into a hospital's management processes, it is not separable from general management.

- *The RM process operates across the organisation.* The RM process can be observed at the level of the individual work set, the sub-unit or the unit. In practice the drive to participate in RM has most often come from unit level, although in some sites the initial stimulus came from the district.

- *For successful implementation the RM process requires: commitment by the relevant personnel; devolution of appropriate authority to the various organisational levels; collaboration between disciplines; managerial support; and appropriate direction from the RM implementation strategy.* Of these elements, commitment was generally high. Devolution of authority was more of a problem in that it required individuals being willing to take on, and surrender, responsibilities. Budgetary devolution was seen as critical. Collaboration was frequently more striking within, than between, disciplines. Many nurses, for example, felt that traditional relationship patterns had not altered. The need for support was recognised, but perhaps not its scale, involving as it did organisational arrangements, data provision, new managerial roles and training. The emphasis in the RM strategy varied between the sites at various times, but over the period of the experiment there was convergence in needing to influence the whole organisation.

- *The adoption of the RM process.* By the end of the study the RM process had, to a greater or lesser extent, been adopted at most sites, notably at the sub-unit or specialty level. This stands as the major achievement of the experiment to date!

E. Resource requirements (see Chapter 5, The Resource Requirements of RM)

- *Costs of RM are difficult to define and to identify.* The resources for RM projects came both from specific additional resources and from reallocation of existing resources, particularly staff time. Although the combined total of these is the true cost, pragmatically this study concentrated on the additional costs of the RM projects. These additional costs include one-off investment cost elements (for example in computer hardware and software) organisation development and staff time involved in implementation.

- *It is unclear whether, for this exercise, the operational ward ordering/reporting systems should be included in the boundary of the costs of RM.* In particular at the two sites where specific Hospital Information Systems have, or are being, implemented, the costs (and benefits) of the two may need to be considered together.

■ *The estimates of additional expenditure on RM (excluding HIS) in the period 1986-87 to 1989-90 ranged from £354,000 to £2.604 million.* The lowest figure is for Arrowe Park which still has to implement its main computer systems. For all other sites the costs are more than double the top of the range of cost estimated in HN(86)34 (viz £400,000 - £600,000).

■ *Although these costs are considerable, taken as an investment over five years, they represent a cost per in-patient episode of between £7.80 and £27.30.* These in turn represent an increase in costs per in-patient episode of between 1.4 and 3.3 per cent.

■ *Estimates of the value of existing resources committed to RM suggest that these figures should be increased by 20-45 per cent to allow for reallocated staff time.*

■ *Including HIS, the additional expenditure was substantially higher.* At the Royal Hampshire, the site where the in-patient element of HIS was completely implemented, the total investment in RM and HIS in the period 1987-88 to 1989-90 was £5.384 million.

■ *The costs of running a 'fully implemented' RM process are still not clear.* Sites are still experimenting with, and learning how to run RM. Moreover, the extent to which RM costs were substitutes for previous management and information costs was unclear. But illustrative examples, particularly of the resources for sub-unit management arrangements, may act as a guide.

F. Benefits of RM (see Chapter 6, Benefits of RM)

■ *The quality of available data on the overall performance of the six sites relative to the national picture is not good enough to make firm comparisons.* The impression is that the six sites may have out-performed the national average on such key indicators as reduction in length of stay.

■ *RM has demonstrated service production benefits.* The research found a number of examples of planned changes in the organisation of services which could logically be attributed to RM and which had increased quality of the service or reduced its cost.

■ *RM can produce benefits in terms of increased service activities.* Examples were found where RM has led to increases in service activity by reallocating resources. But some examples suggest that RM has led to a decrease in activity.

■ *RM may or may not produce benefits to patient care.* No measurable improvements in patient care were found, although some of the service production changes were seen by patients as improving the delivery of care.

- *Doctors and nurses remain broadly positive about RM.* There was a wide spectrum of perceptions of the value of RM but, in general, service providers did not feel that RM had yet produced significant benefits. It is striking that even after four years experience of RM, the majority appeared to believe that benefits could still be realised in the future. This belief was tempered by perceptions of the opportunity costs represented by the financial and other resource implications associated with RM.

- *Key managers saw RM as having significantly helped the units to manage change.* They believed the key features of RM were now robust elements of the management of the units. None would wish to go back to more traditional ways of managing.

- *It is still too early to expect to see the full benefits of the computer technology.* Implementation of computer systems is not yet complete, a time-lag before benefits are achieved is inevitable.

LESSONS FROM THE RM INITIATIVE

Not unusually one of the major sub-plots of the book is that the world of the NHS has not stood still. The detailed objectives and expectations of RM at the pilot sites have been adjusted as the context has changed. The nature of the management framework has been radically altered by the move to contracting as from April 1991, and so the use of RM and its value to the hospital organisation has been changed. In many ways the RM Initiative was an attempt to achieve cultural change within hospitals without changing their external managerial and financial relationships. The objectives of RM were to encourage greater efficiency, to persuade clinicians to be involved in management, to facilitate the provision of data linking resources to clinical activity, and to foster an environment where resources could be actively managed to achieve desired change in patient services.

The White Paper has effectively changed the circumstances so that such changes are now more and more essential to organisational success rather than simply desirable for the 'social good' they can do. Thus rather than needing convincing about the benefits of RM, 130 units are already part of the formal process of 'roll out', others are making independent moves towards RM, and the concerns from the medical profession about doctors in management have diminished.

Given these changes, it might appear that this evaluation is merely rather inconclusive documentation of an interesting, but now largely irrelevant, step in the development of NHS management. For each of the six sites involvement in the RM

Initiative has been a catalyst for major cultural change. They have learnt from their early mistakes and successes, and have shown that learning process in the way they have adapted and adjusted their process of implementation, changing emphases, reassessing priorities and revising plans. Many of the lessons they have learnt individually may be quite specific to their particular circumstances and not readily generalisable (Coombs *et al.*, 1991).

However, there are a number of important lessons for the future that emerge from the research that do seem to have wider relevance. These 'lessons' fall into three main groups: for other acute units at early stages in the implementation of RM; for the central health policy-makers (the Department of Health and the NHS Management Executive) in establishing similar policy initiatives; and for those concerned to try to evaluate broad managerial changes such as RM.

Lessons for sites embarking on RM

Other sites embarking on RM will, no doubt, each draw their own rather different set of lessons from the experiences of the six, but our research evidence suggests that they should all consider the following issues:

- *It is necessary to understand what RM really is.* RM is primarily about cultural change, with providers actively moving to a role where they are involved in planning their services, and managing the resources they and colleagues commit to achieve agreed plans. It involves accepting responsibility for coping with difficult circumstances rather than laying the responsibility elsewhere. It involves collaboration. It has implications for all levels and parts of the organisation and for all professional groups. Computer technology is subsidiary to this. If cultural change cannot be achieved, RM will not succeed.

- *If RM is to work, it has to become (the major) part of the normal process of the management of the hospital.* Its development and implementation need to be positively and vigorously encouraged and supported by the UGM (or chief executive). This means, not least, that in decentralising responsibility, the UGM and central management function of the hospital has to be willing to devolve power. RM is not a bolt-on optional extra.

- *The key to a successful RM process is the development of a strong sub-unit organisation* with service providers being given and accepting budgetary responsibility within a framework of agreed service plans. The concept of a clinical directorate is the clearest form of such decentralised responsibility, but other variants are possible providing there is unambiguous focus, with proactive clinical leadership. This sub-unit organisation will need management support, including a financial management input; and regular appropriate routine data on activities, budgets and manpower systems, together with facilities for the easy handling of non-routine data requests.

■ The experience of the RM Initiative sites confirms the well-known but nevertheless often forgotten rule that an information strategy needs to precede and underlay decisions about data collection and information technology. *There needs to be a clear vision of who is to manage, what is to be managed, and how the process of management will take place.* In practice this will be an evolutionary process as, with use, data needs are more clearly defined and information flows refined to reflect need. But computer systems are not so flexible that the process of data collection can start without a clear and carefully articulated initial vision of the future management process.

■ The magnitude and multifaceted nature of RM means that *there is a dangerous tendency to allow development of the process, particularly of the development of information systems, to take place in a fragmented manner.* Data in feeder systems from support departments, nursing information and clinical information all have to play a role in the collaborative management of resources. They have to satisfy immediate operational management needs and longer-term strategic planning needs.

■ *It is essential that key groups are not marginalised or left to work in isolation.* Individual professions have to meet their specific management needs but more importantly contribute to the needs of the professional group concerned and of the overall management of resources. Some of the concerns about the development of nurse management information systems may stem from the fact that these have sometimes been developed in a degree of professional isolation.

■ *The establishment of the necessary ownership of the information used for management is necessary, is hard, and is only slowly achieved.* Users need to understand and accept ownership of the data definitions, of the data collection systems, and of the data analysis. Only slowly will the computer be believed in preference to the traditional system and for many months the former is likely to be checked against manual records.

■ *Do not underestimate the development and training needs.* Even in a project such as RM Initiative, where the organisational development and training needs were recognised, they were still underestimated. All sites repeatedly found the need to intensify training and to consolidate the understanding of developments, before proceeding further.

■ *Implementation projects such as RM require a substantial element of project planning*, encompassing not just the processes relating to computer system implementation (specifications, procurement, installation, testing, etc.) but also the elements of organisational change and of the inputs of organisational development and training. Planning should incorporate clear and definable milestones to monitor progress and these again should not just concern computer systems. If it is to serve as a tool for managing and monitoring the project and to act as an encouragement to those struggling to achieve the plans, planning needs to be realistic and not just optimistic.

■ *Ideally, the planning of change involves maintaining old systems until the new systems can take over.* Several of the sites have suffered from periods when flows of basic information have deteriorated or ceased altogether, when existing systems have been stopped before new systems have been fully operational. Parallel working of systems may be expensive or in some cases impossible, but the result of not doing so will be a period without even the previous level of information. At worst this may cause, for example, a financial crisis, or less dramatically it may simply reduce the credibility of the route to better management.

Lessons for central policy initiatives

From a policy perspective, RM is one of a series of initiatives concerned with improving the management of the public sector. As such, many of the problems encountered in the RM Initiative have relevance to similar initiatives in the future.

■ *The choice of an approach that 'pilots' an initiative in local sites, where there are evident preconditions for success and vigorous and powerful local champions, clearly has advantages.* It provides a test under conditions that give the initiative a real chance, and minimises the chance of sites falling by the wayside when the road is long and at times hard. It is remarkable that five of the original six sites identified in HN(86)34 have stuck with the process and achieved so much (and that the original sixth, Clatterbridge, is effectively back on board as part of Wirral Hospital after a period of major structural change). However, that approach has meant a loss of central control over the way in which RM has been implemented. Initial diversity in approach has had both advantages and disadvantages. The research team observed a very strong tendency towards convergence of thinking on many issues, particularly on organisational arrangements - convergence greater in reality than some of the rhetoric of the individual sites might suggest.

■ Partly as a result of the different local agendas the initiative had a variety of objectives. *Common objectives were really so broad that their achievement was hard to assess, and even harder to measure objectively.* There was no focal attempt to set out the nature of the new management process in specific terms and to identify the linkage between the broad subsidiary process objectives, of involving doctors and nurses in management and providing them with appropriate management information, and the primary objective of achieving measurable improvements of patient care.

In the original Health Notice, the one quantified target of releasing one percent of annual expenditure for redeployment on patient services, represented a difference that would almost inevitably be lost in the noise of changes in hospital costs and activity rates due to a whole range of other real factors, and in apparent changes due to differences in methods of cost measurement or definition.

- *The likelihood of measuring the impact of RM was greatly reduced by the rapidity of subsequent, and in many ways more fundamental, changes* in NHS organisation and management brought about by the NHS Review. Whilst clearly the pace of reform has to be determined by political factors, the extent to which the NHS can learn from pilot initiatives such as this is vastly diminished, if the pace is such that reforms follow each other without an intervening opportunity to assess their independent impact.

- *With hindsight the original initiative was grossly optimistic both about timescales and the costs of RM.* Guidance in the initial circular announcing RM suggested development costs in the range £400,000 to £600,000 per site, of which 70 per cent would be met from central funds. Our evidence from the sites indicated that over the period 1987-88 to 1990-91, the central contribution was three times that estimated.   At the end of 1990 the Financial Management Executive was suggesting that each new hospital participating in RM could expect to receive around £1 million for development over three years (NHS Management Executive, 1990).   Some optimism may have been necessary to encourage participation, but the over-optimism in this case may well have been in part responsible for loss of momentum at many of the sites in 1989-1990, when, three years into the project, even the more committed participants were realising that there was still a long way to go to achieve their goals.

- Slower progress than anticipated was in part due to shortages of key skills within the service, and lack of relevant experience in some suppliers. These skills were exacerbated by the roll-out plans which led to the diffusion of many key personnel from the pilot sites, especially project managers, to other NHS units and, more particularly, to the private sector consultants. *Even more central attention has to be paid to the availability of the real resources needed, not just to financial support.*

■ The pilot sites were the focus of considerable attention and interest. In addition to a regular and heavy flow of visitors from elsewhere in the NHS they drew political and media attention. It appears that this limelight had its benefits initially, in encouraging a local pride in what was being done and a healthy competitive spirit between the sites, but after a time the burden of laying on regular tours, of key personnel speaking at seminars etc., began to take its toll. The RM unit provided some support latterly but *the sites would have benefited if the educational aspect of the 'pilot initiative' had been more consciously planned for and resources earmarked for this role.*

■ *Clear central leadership is needed to maintain cohesiveness and momentum.* Initially, leadership of the Initiative was very visible, with a very positive involvement of the then Director of Finance, regular meetings of the Chairmen of each local steering group with the central team, and regular attendance of RM officials at local steering group meetings. Over time and with the change in director of finance this top-level central leadership diminished, and the cohesiveness that it had generated dissipated. The six sites began to feel that central attention had turned firmly to the roll-out sites, which they also felt, rightly or wrongly, were in many cases being treated financially more favourably. This, too, may have exacerbated the loss of momentum, and is a factor that deserves more careful attention in future initiatives.

Lessons for evaluation

The RM Initiative was unusual in terms of the explicit commitment to evaluation in the original circular, in part the result of the agreement with the JCC. The decision to go ahead with independent evaluation has to be applauded. Hopefully this evaluation, however imperfect, justifies the decision to evaluate. If evaluation is to be undertaken in future, this case study points to a number of general issues that need to be taken on board:

■ A problem from the start was that the evaluation began after the beginning of the RM Initiative, permitting the researchers no opportunity to get a true base-line assessment of the hospitals. This, in itself, inevitably led to a greater focus on the process of implementation. And, effectively, the research ended before implementation was complete. To extend the period of research would probably have simply reduced its usefulness to central and local policy-makers. *In future the period of evaluation will need to be planned more realistically, to start earlier before intervention and to continue to an agreed point of policy completion.*

■ *A fundamental problem in evaluating change of this sort is the absence of specific controls.* The proposed triangulation methodology, comparing the effects of RM within participating sites and with non-participating sites (see Appendix 1), appeared to offer a partial solution to the problem, but in the event was less successful than had been hoped. The main reasons for the lack of success were (i) the major changes occurring generally in the NHS and the adoption of aspects of the RM by many sites; (ii) the still enormous problem in getting comparable data on performance of the sites themselves and of the NHS as a whole; (iii) the convergence of the approaches at the sites so that comparisons between them were less helpful than might have been the case. In terms of the latter point, it might have been better to recruit two small groups of sites, each group committed to undertaking RM in a different way (for example: with or without major computer system investment) to provide a clearer internal comparison.

■ The research approach adopted was summative rather than formative - to observe and record independently rather than to try to influence the process of implementation. *A summative approach still seems most appropriate given the context of this evaluation, but it raises problems of incentives to the sites to actively co-operate.* In practice, access and help from many at the sites was exemplary but there were problems in maintaining adequate contact with all aspects of RM, and in maintaining the necessary commitment from the sites; problems made worse by the changes in key RM staff from which most of the sites suffered. Incentives for commitment to such research need to be considered more directly in future.

■ There is a more general problem, alluded to above, in that attempts to improve the quality of data available in the NHS to measure hospital performance make the process of comparison in the short-term even more difficult. National changes, such as the introduction of Körner data systems, and local changes to new computer systems, each create gaps and discontinuities, which completely overwhelm many of the changes it is wished to measure. *Greater statistical continuity is needed if any meaningful evaluation, independent or internal, is to be possible.*

■ *There is an inherent problem in evaluating management policies that are aimed in a general sense at improving patient care, but do not specifically incorporate measures for determining whether such improvement is taking place.* The 'hands-off' approach adopted in this study had a high danger of ending with an unproven verdict with respect to improvements, simply because adequate measures did not exist at the sites. However, to set these up as part of the research measuring systems, which inevitably cannot be independent of the hospital information systems, alters the very nature of the management intervention that is being evaluated. Thus returning to the first lesson for the future sites, measurable objectives need to be agreed and the necessary means to measure them set up as an integral part of the initiatives.

THE BALANCE OF EVIDENCE

At a point almost exactly four years after the announcement of the RM Initiative, it is still not possible to provide a definitive assessment of RM as an on-going working process for hospital management.

In terms of implementation, it can be definitively asserted that the original timescale envisaged in HN(86)34 was unrealistic: the sites still have some way to go before they each have a complete RM system in place and RM has fully become the routine of hospital management. Progress has been slow and patchy as predicted by Pollitt *et al.*, (1988). Thus, this study has observed implementation, rather than implementation followed by a period of established use.

Progress may have been slower than anticipated but substantial progress towards full implementation has been, and continues to be, made at each of the sites, despite all the other pressures upon them. None of the sites have given up or decided that RM is not worthwhile. Indeed, perhaps the most striking evidence is the conviction of key managers at the six sites, that it has been worthwhile and that they would not want to go back to managing in the traditional way. Much has been learnt in the process, of value not only to the original six, but to others following in their wake, not least that RM involves a major cultural change for the whole organisation.

Although implementation may not be complete, elements of the RM process have firmly taken root at all sites. Particularly at the sub-unit level there has been a major change towards more proactive management by service providers. What is more, our research concludes that there is a strong internal logic to RM. RM resolves long standing problems of the NHS in respect of enabling service activities to be genuinely managed, rather than having their management divided between resource allocation and patient care. Collaboration amongst service providers, and between service providers and management is promoted. Authority and accountability for decisions about the allocation of resources, their management and the planning and review of services, are combined into a coherent whole. It should also be noted that this internal logic in entirely compatible with approaches to strengthen service management and improve the quality of care advocated in the NHS Review.

The study found that the attitudes to RM of doctors and nurses at the sites was generally positive towards RM, although still expecting greater benefits than had so far been experienced. In terms of the questions to clinicians posed in the Annex to the original Health Notice, the picture that emerges from the study is summarised in Box 7.1. The responses range from the positive view about clinicians being involved, to a rather partial success as regards data, through to an agnostic but still hopeful view as to the balance of time versus benefit.

But again in the specific terms of the Notice, RM cannot yet be said to have produced a system that has demonstrated its ability to achieve significant measurable patient benefits. There are assertions of improvements in patient care and we have indicated examples of these where the link to RM as a causal factor seems justifiable but, in a health service generally striving to make such improvements, it is difficult to prove that they would not have happened without RM. As to the release of 1 per cent of expenditure for redeployment, it is quite feasible that this has happened, but impossible to isolate in the statistics.

Despite this, there is good reason to conclude positively about the value of the management processes and organisational structures associated with RM. And once the transition has been achieved there is little reason to suppose that these need add significantly to the real unit management costs.

But the case for the relatively expensive infrastructure of computer technology remains open. Many of the examples of service benefits that have been noted have not stemmed from improved information but from the ability to agree a strategy and to implement that strategy; whereas previously the solution had been well known but no action had been feasible. Hospitals have many existing sources of information not captured on computers - not least the knowledge and experience in people's heads. Highly sophisticated data is not needed to change admission times, or to reorganise use of theatres; but these do need a managerial context in which they can be addressed, decisions made, and acted upon. There is, of course, a logic that improved data will improve decisions further but the evidence from the RM Initiative is that the benefits of improved data (and by extension the benefits of the systems that produce it) are slower to emerge.

Several sites do see their computer systems as being a major competitive asset in the world of NHS contracting; and indeed some of the computer technology associated with RM may be very advantageous in this context, but that is not to say that it is clearly a beneficial part of the process of getting doctors and nurses successfully involved in management. The computers may yield benefits when clinicians as part of a broad concept of audit are regularly able to review their workload in terms of an acceptable categorisation of case mix, comparing their resource use and success rates with those of colleagues within their own hospital and further afield. But that particular vision is still some way off.

For the present each of these six sites has moved a long way towards a management process that enables service providers to be actively involved in the

Box 7.1 Tests for the success of RM

1. Has the management scheme involved fully the clinicians?

Broadly, yes.

2. Has this enabled the clinicians to have a positive influence on the management of resources of the unit?

Yes, but still limited by the scope to change traditional power structures.

3. Have the information systems provided data relevant to patient care and has the information been of value to clinicians in providing that care?

Data has been provided patchily to sub-units and individuals. To date value has been limited.

4. What have been the direct and indirect costs of implementing the scheme and have these costs been justified by the resulting benefits of the scheme?

Direct costs were higher than estimated. Indirect costs of implementation were high but were largely absorbed. No evidence yet that costs have been matched by benefits.

5. Has the time-input required by clinicians to implement the scheme been considered by the clinicians themselves to be beneficial to patient care?

Consultants remain agnostic on this question, although still anticipating future benefits.

management of the resources they commit, with computer systems that should support that process. Benefits are beginning to emerge and the potential almost certainly exists to use RM to improve the efficiency or quality of care to more than cover the small (1-4 per cent) increase in cost per case that the RM investment has added. But that potential requires positive realisation.

Finally, it could fairly be asked whether in 1986 the time for RM had indeed come? Has the experience of the RM Initiative demonstrated any success in advancing the four policy-related elements which, it was suggested in Chapter 1, constituted RM?

- *Improved quality of care.* This remained as the motivation, the hope that encouraged many of the service providers to participate in RM. As has been indicated above, there is some evidence that RM has been of direct benefit to patients, but it is slender and not particularly conclusive. There is rather more confidence from the service that, given more time, RM can improve quality of care. Certainly where information on their activities has been available, service providers have examined it with interest and considered, if often sceptically, if there were lessons to be learned. A few also commenced devising and testing outcome measures. By 1991 'quality' has come to be a fashionable issue, with attention directed to audit, to quality assurance as part of the contractual system and to the Total Quality Management experiments. The RM Initiative has contributed to this emphasis. Certainly the use of information on activities in monitoring and evaluating services is basic to the RM process.

- *Involvement in management by the service providers.* The RM Initiative does appear to bring the service providers and general managers closer together. Although the participation of service providers has been uneven, overall they have been drawn more into managing their resources and general managers have devolved some of their authority to sub-units or individuals. Indeed some form or other of sub-unit organisational structure appears as a necessary basis for service providers to manage the application of resources to patient care. Overall, the connection between clinical activity and resource use has become less controversial (Coombs *et al.*, 1991). However integration and mutual understanding are not the only possible scenarios. Some service providers still fear RM as a decoy, intended to subordinate their clinical freedom through tighter control of costs and activities and the imposition of a managerial hierarchy. A rather different vision is of increasing medical power; with clinicians using the RM process and clinical directorates to assume managerial control.

- *Improved information.* The sites participating in the RM Initiative have undoubtedly, and not without some trauma, been brought closer to the mainstream of modern institutional practice. Where information was available it was welcomed and used but computer systems took longer than was initially envisaged to be installed and operational, in that a direct translation from commercial, or foreign health service, applications was rarely possible. But looking more widely, the NHS still appears to be lagging behind other comparable organisations in making use of information technology (National Audit Office, 1990). Indeed from the standpoint of competing within a market, one critical view is that the NHS record of investment is:

> light years behind most of commerce and business of a comparable
> size and complexity (Prowle *et al.*, 1989).

This is not necessarily fatal for RM. Improved information is a product of new processes and relationships; for example, resulting from an orientation towards service outputs through sub-unit structures, and does not have to depend upon complex computer systems.

■ *Stronger control of resources.* The relationship between service supporters (the tax payers and politicians), the service givers and the service recipients is essentially unchanged by RM. RM remains controlled by the service givers although, as suggested above, there may have been internal adjustments between different interests within the NHS. RM does potentially give the service supporters a clearer view as to where the resources are going, but part of the motivation for service providers, in particular, to engage in RM, is the increased ability it gives them to justify their view of resource needs. Resources have been strongly controlled over the period of the experiment but this has owed more to traditional strategies, such as tight, cash limited budgets and service reviews, which have not necessarily been applied in accordance with the principles of RM. Indeed the latter has generally sought to play-down the costing aspects. With the NHS Review, the government turned to other, market orientated means of controlling resources.

When this evaluation commenced, in 1988, commentators on the NHS were already suggesting that the factors influencing the success of RM might all:

> be affected by a radical restructuring of the NHS (Pollitt *et al.*, 1988).

At the time of writing this book the NHS is indeed in the process of being 'radically restructured'. The NHS Review changed the incentives for RM. As Prowle and his colleagues (1989) warn, hospitals:

need to take considerable care when undertaking RM Initiative projects to ensure that the developments are consistent with the future local needs required to meet the demands of *Working for Patients*.

So the potential for RM to advance its constituent elements depends now upon how it is used within the wider context of the new NHS.

THE ORGANISATION TRANSFORMED

INTRODUCTION

In 1986, RM was a collection of ideas which six sites were charged with understanding and integrating into their existing activities. Those involved had in effect to invent RM, and it was perhaps inevitable that as time went on their understanding of it, and hence their ambitions for it, changed. In the preceding chapters, it has been made clear that no site has yet fully developed RM: in particular, those which have made most progress still retain a large measure of central control, and have devolved authority only patchily.

There is no single, shared vision of RM either within or between sites. Yet several people at the sites, notably some of those who have been most closely involved in developing RM, retain a vision of a way of managing services which has not yet been achieved. The visions of these individuals are by no means identical, reflecting differences in local circumstances and personal interests, but they share a common core of ideas. In this chapter we draw on these ideas to articulate our own vision, and consider the nature of an organisation transformed by RM.

It would, in principle, be possible here to emphasise any of a number of characteristics of the organisation, but we have elected to focus on just a few. Some, such as collaboration and devolution of authority have been introduced in earlier chapters: others, such as the role of information are discussed for the first time.

COLLABORATION, AUTHORITY AND CONTROL

RM builds on several of the most positive characteristics exhibited by the pilot sites. The most important of these are the willingness to collaborate across professional boundaries, and the alignment of authority and accountability for the allocation of resources. Their effects can be traced by looking at three areas where collaboration already occurs. Collaboration does not imply that people have to have identical objectives: rather, they can have their own, reflecting their particular interests, but they must agree on those that most affect all involved parties.

The first category of collaboration is that between general managers and consultants and other service providers, the activity most closely associated with RM. An instructive way of examining the issue is to look at changes in the nature of control systems used within the hospital. In most NHS hospitals, control is principally financial and exercised unilaterally at unit level. With RM, in contrast, there are interlocking control systems, operated at sub-unit level. The task of the unit is to co-ordinate and integrate activities at sub-unit level. At unit level, resources are allocated as part of the annual planning cycle: the key task is to plan services so as to achieve the best trade-off between activity, cost and quality. These are formalised each year into specific objectives in discussion with sub-units, and service delivery is monitored against them.

To some extent, processes at sub-unit level reflect those at unit level; but the sub-unit is now the hub of the organisation. RM involves two transformations: from an organisation based on a division of labour to one based on division of knowledge; and from top-down to distributed control. Together, these transformations mean that decisions are made closer to the points of service delivery, and the organisation is focused towards patients. The difference between this and traditional financial control can hardly be overstated. Service providers must work together towards objectives that they have helped to set: if they pull in different directions control cannot be exercised properly.

Control has also to be integrated with that being exercised in other sub-units: this is achieved in part at unit level but is also effected directly between sub-units. The information needed to exercise control cannot be solely financial, but must span activity, cost and quality, which are in some way linked. Distributed control requires explicit trade-offs across the three dimensions.

Together, these points highlight the importance of collaboration, since sub-units are typically fairly small groupings which cannot work if people do not agree to work towards common goals. RM improves decision-making by bringing together the best people to take decisions, one of the most important of which is sub-unit groupings. Since decisions are not always palatable, collaboration helps to ensure that people share in taking unpopular decisions: at least the process of taking such decisions is more civilised. Authority is also important because without it sub-units will not be able to exercise effective control over resource use. This is not to say that all authority should be devolved to sub-units, but only that for which service providers are particularly qualified and can be expected to take accountability: that is, for clinical decision-making. Authority for other decisions can be retained elsewhere.

The combination of collaboration and devolution of authority implies major differences in the power structures with RM compared to those usually found in NHS hospitals. Commentators on RM have highlighted the involvement of clinicians in general management processes, implying that they are drawn into a hierarchical structure. But the irony is that the hierarchy of the new organisation is strictly limited, a consequence of the focus on sub-units. Service providers operate at all levels of the organisation, blurring hierarchical distinctions. The price of RM for both managers and service providers is a loss of power in certain areas, this being compensated for by sharing power (i.e. gaining power) over a greater range of activities than before.

One characteristic of an organisation with distributed control is that it is, at least in principle, more flexible and hence responsive to internal and external change. RM thus offers a route from the hierarchical organisation of the past, which was suited to a relatively stable environment, to an organisation better suited to a world of rapid change and greater uncertainty (Burns and Stalker, 1966). The limited hierarchy, with strong horizontal links, suggests that many staff will have a span of knowledge far greater than their spans of authority or control. This is most obvious in the role of the sub-unit business manager, who at present is expected to have a broad knowledge of the organisation, but often lacks the authority to obtain that knowledge, notably about nursing activities. The transformed organisation makes sense of the business manager's role: the differences in the spans are in fact natural and inevitable. The key difference is that with distributed control the imperatives to share information are greater.

Clarification of the responsibility of sub-units for control of resource use highlights an important paradox. The information collected in order to monitor services is intended to do two things. One of these is to provide the information to allow control to be exercised. In many organisations control tends to be unilateral, its purpose being to ensure that people are behaving 'according to plan'. The controlled individuals thus have their activities opened up to scrutiny, and this can result in them adopting strategies to avoid its consequences. However, the same information is intended to be used by service providers to review - i.e. learn about - their own work. The threat or actual imposition of control may lead to them failing or refusing to learn from the information provided. So control and learning may be opposed to one another. By devolving control, RM seeks to resolve this paradox, since control and learning are aligned: they are performed by the same people.

Indeed, a major risk in the design of (manual or computerised) information systems is that they can be used to reinforce the status quo. In principle, computers can produce information in ways which support new practices or reinforce old ones. Basic decisions about what data is to be stored on them, who will have access to what data, and above all who has authority to change entries, can become immutable features of the system design. The aim must be to use them to automate activities, provide information for decision-making, and thus help transform the organisation.

The second area where collaboration is important comes under the general rubric of service review, involving both different professional groups and members of a single profession in monitoring and evaluation of services. Service review orients discussions explicitly towards patients, and concerns providing the highest quality of care possible. The organisation is thus balanced between control and a focus on care processes. These processes also take place at sub-unit level, though in separate meetings to those concerned with allocation of resources. Service review is thus a subset of RM: distinct from it, but sharing several of its characteristics. The objectives of the two are also complementary, both being concerned with the effectiveness of service delivery. Accordingly, service review should be linked directly into unit and directorate management. A separate reporting structure would only confuse arrangements for reporting to the management board, whereas with the processes linked a sub-unit could present a single, coherent picture to the rest of the organisation.

Processes at sub-unit level can be thought of as dealing with a spectrum of issues, with rationing at one end and good practice at the other. Over time each has broadened its scope along the spectrum, so that the two overlap. RM incorporates explicit consideration of quality, as service review incorporates the resource implications of service delivery. But this elision is not without its dangers, the most crucial of which is the possibility of management interference in clinical practice. This is an ethical issue, which requires service providers to rethink their views on clinical freedom, and merits constant monitoring.

The organisation with RM is different only in the pervasiveness of discussion: it is part of the culture. The rationale for discussion here is that it results in better decisions about care delivery than those taken by individuals acting alone. (This might be a statement of the obvious, were it not for the general interpretation of clinical freedom which implies that individual doctors could and should act alone in many situations.) Such discussions do carry a time cost, and in many cases there is no particular need to consult: but discussion is perceived to be intrinsically valuable, both for service providers and patients, and so is commonplace.

The focus on computers in RM has led many people to assume that they must be the organisation's principal source of information. This assumption is wrong: the organisation is a sea of information, only some of which is captured by computers. Indeed, this seems rather obvious once realised: medical records are rich sources, and what about all the information in people's heads which underlies their expertise?

The collection and use of information is perhaps more intensively concentrated in hospitals than almost any other type of organisation, and the average level of formal education of staff is very high. But while many staff are highly educated, there nevertheless exist natural 'information asymmetries' between professional groups, due to differences in training and in work experience. Nurses know things that doctors don't and vice versa. These asymmetries can be a source of communication difficulties between groups, but can also be viewed positively if people are willing to communicate in order to reduce the asymmetries: they can pool their knowledge to improve decision-making. Sharing information - whether of the sort contained in a medical record, or 'general' knowledge available only to a particular group - helps to reduce (though not eliminate) asymmetries permanently.

It is the promise of improvements in the quality of decision-making which provides much of the rationale for collaboration between individuals at all levels of the organisation. But there are two important pre-requisites for communication across boundaries. The first of these is that people trust one another. It might seem obvious that trust is important - it is in any relationship - but it has seldom been recognised as such in organisations in the NHS. Trust must operate both vertically and horizontally. It underpins the devolution of authority to directorates and wards and departments and to individuals. And it characterises relationships within and between directorates.

The emphasis on collaboration should not blind us to the importance of individuals in RM. The RM process starts and ends with individuals. It is individuals who experience cultural changes and elect to work in new ways. Consultants, for example, will carry a particular set of predispositions with them as they go onto wards or spend time reviewing their work, which will influence the decisions they make.

By implication, people on either side of these professional and disciplinary boundaries understand something of the world of the other. That is, they have developed a cognitive model of the organisation which is no longer based only on their own immediate sphere of interest, but extends into other parts of the organisation. This in turn encourages a sense of belonging, of ownership. Collaborative working practices are widespread, with the result that people working on opposite sides of organisational and professional boundaries can understand the value of information to others, and that much information is of benefit to both sides. For example, nursing and medical records staff agree that information on patient movement is important both for operational management and for understanding longer term trends.

The second pre-requisite for collaboration is a 'language' for communication across professional boundaries. Candidates for such a language have been proposed in the past, including Körner data (DHSS, 1982-84) and DRGs (Bardsley *et al.*, 1987). To date, neither of these has made a convincing claim, although work continues on DRG-type grouping of cases. There are, though, a number of types of information which are generally understood and can be widely discussed.

It is useful to distinguish here between a 'common language' and a 'shared language'. Common languages are designed to be used by everyone when talking about a given domain, irrespective of their background. Shared languages, in contrast, may be more exclusive, and used only by small groups of staff. Thus doctors and nurses within a specialty may develop a shared language for communication about local issues. RM is about the development of both types of language.

The types of collaboration described above are concerned with making the organisation inherently flexible. The final area examined here is concerned with developing the organisation. Clearly, different types of development require different people to come together, and these may be temporary alliances within the organisation, or alliances with outside parties. The rationale for these alliances is both practical and political, being concerned with bringing together the people who can get the job done and in avoiding or overcoming opposition within the organisation.

Even the best organisations can develop within them a variety of strategies for avoiding change, and temporary alliances can be useful devices for overcoming them. Many of the characteristics of RM discussed earlier also apply to the change process. Those involved must have authority devolved to them, they must set clear objectives, and so on.

Perhaps the most important point here is that there is ultimately no boundary between the implementation phase and the transformed organisation. RM is an evolutionary process with no end-point. This means that implementation is as much a part of RM as the process: so *how* it is implemented determines whether or not the organisation can be transformed. It is not possible to implement poorly yet end up with a satisfactory process.

THE EXTERNAL ENVIRONMENT

RM can never be a utopian concept. By its nature it must be part of an imperfect world, where organisations are presented with opportunities and threats from without and within, to which they must respond. Since RM is an integral part of the organisation, it cannot exist in isolation from the world around it. The transformed organisation is patient-oriented, with authority devolved to sub-units: necessarily, priorities are set locally. But the NHS is a centrally-managed organisation, with resources allocated from the top down. Directives, including the NHS Review, arrive from the centre and managers have little choice but to respond: so priorities are also set centrally. The future success of RM depends to a large extent on who determines service priorities. If they are in large part determined centrally, service providers may well become frustrated because they find they are constrained in their discretion over the allocation of resources. At best they will use RM perversely, simply as a way of controlling resource use. Accordingly, if RM is to work, those who determine the allocation of resources must at least be responsive to the arguments put forward by hospitals, and undertake a dialogue using a shared language.

Contracting may eventually complement RM here, by clarifying who allocates resources and how they are to be allocated. But this implies that resource allocation decisions will be made by purchasing authorities, and not by unit management. Sub-units, as holders of contracts, may thrive, but their principal dialogue will then be with purchasers.

This illustrates the more general point about the NHS Review that it changes the incentives for both managers and service providers. Consultant contracts increase the incentives to become involved in management, medical audit for them to review their work. Nurses will in many places be explicitly responsible for planning and monitoring service quality. Managers have a new agenda which places a premium on good information, and requires them to make trade-offs between patient services, capital and (in some cases) newly-flexible staff pay. The new incentives need to be consistent with RM if the latter is to be worthwhile.

Appendix 1

METHODOLOGY AND METHODS

COMMISSIONING OF THE RESEARCH

The RM Initiative was formally announced in HN(86)34 in November 1986. The Health Notice named six acute hospital pilot sites and outlined the aims and objectives which they would seek to achieve. It also stated that the introduction of RM at the pilot sites would be evaluated.

In mid-1986 the Health Economics Research Group (HERG) at Brunel University had indicated its interest in evaluating the costs and benefits of RM at the six pilot sites. An outline proposal was put to the DHSS in late 1986, and a brief feasibility study carried out between April and June 1987. The project was finally commissioned by the Department's Research Management Division in early 1988, and HERG commenced work in May of that year.

This evaluation was to be based on work at each of the six sites listed below:

Royal Hampshire County Hospital, Winchester HA,
Freeman Hospital, Newcastle HA,
Guy's Hospital, Lewisham and North Southwark HA,
Huddersfield Royal Infirmary, Huddersfield HA,
Wirral (Arrowe Park) Hospital, Wirral HA,
Pilgrim Hospital, South Lincolnshire HA.

This list differs in two respects from the list in HN(86)34. First, the Health Notice named two sites in Wirral HA, Clatterbridge and Arrowe Park Hospitals. As a result of uncertainty over its future, Clatterbridge withdrew from the Initiative in 1988. Subsequently however, in late 1989 Clatterbridge was amalgamated with Arrowe Park to form a single management unit, Wirral DGH. The HERG team had earlier elected not to include Clatterbridge in the evaluation, and in spite of the amalgamation decided to focus only on developments at Arrowe Park. Although Clatterbridge was once again part of the RM Initiative, it was felt that there would be insufficient time to arrive at a proper judgement about developments at that site. The second difference is that the Pilgrim Hospital was not listed in the Health Notice, but was formally adopted as a RM site in April 1988 and has been included in this evaluation.

The Notice also named thirteen community units which would participate in RM. In contrast to the acute hospital sites, the community units were described as *demonstration* sites. There had been two pilot community units, Bromley and Worcester, in the earlier Management Budgeting initiative, and these had been judged a success by the Department. Thus the thirteen new sites were to build on the success of the first two, and were deemed not to require evaluation. Accordingly, no attempt was made to evaluate the community sites, and they are not discussed in this book.

RESEARCH METHODS

Initially the principal purpose of the evaluation was to establish whether or not the RM Initiative resulted in measurable improvements in patient care. This is in line with HN(86)34, whose principal objective was:

> the introduction of a new approach to resource management and to demonstrating whether or not this results in measurable improvements in patient care (DHSS, 1986a).

The evaluation was thus concerned principally with the Initiative as a whole; that is, with the totality of the experiences of the six sites rather than with evaluating each one individually. It was clear from the outset that obtaining an understanding of the impact of RM would require a detailed review of each of the six sites. The feasibility study and the research proposal agreed with the (then) DHSS highlighted the importance of observing directly the experiences of six very different sites in implementing RM. The proposal reflected the tension that typically arises in policy evaluations between the needs of policy makers and researchers, who operate to different timescales. Policy makers often operate to relatively short timescales, and have to frame new policies on the basis of political imperatives and incomplete information regarding existing initiatives, whereas researchers always seek the ideal of waiting until an initiative is fully implemented and its effects observed, before making any judgements. The approach to the research outlined here represents a compromise between the two positions. Given the resources available, it was agreed that the evaluation should comprise similar work at all six sites but focus on two, the Royal Hampshire County and Freeman Hospitals. At these two sites, the research would concentrate further on two specialties. It was subsequently agreed that in order to reflect the growing emphasis on RM at sub-unit level, a single specialty would also be identified and its progress reviewed at the other four sites.

The first monitoring phase of the study was undertaken between May 1988 and April 1989, and an Interim Report was published in July 1989 (Buxton *et al.*, 1989). The principal focus was on the progress made by the six pilot sites in implementing RM, and a strategy was devised to obtain a general view of developments. This involved interviews, attendance at meetings, and obtaining documentation describing the sites' current status and future plans. As part of this process, agreement was reached with the general surgeons and physicians at the Royal Hampshire and the Freeman to provide our 'case studies' at the sub-unit level. Additionally, at each of the other four sites, one clinician or sub-unit agreed to provide the researchers with access to their work.

In addition to the work at the hospitals, developments occurring at national level and more widely in the NHS were monitored. The most important single development, the NHS Review, was published only a few months prior to the Interim Report.

After the publication of the Interim Report, the research followed two tracks. The first was to continue monitoring the pilot sites: the first phase of the work had established that none of the sites had yet fully implemented RM, and it was deemed important to continue to monitor progress with implementation. The second track concerned the evaluation of the six sites in terms of the costs and benefits of RM.

The methodological basis of the research rested initially on a number of assumptions about RM, namely that:

- it would be fully implemented at the sites during the course of the study, and that it would be possible to monitor a full year's use of RM in the period from April 1989. At the very least, quantitative data from new information systems would be available to facilitate analysis of the impact of RM;

- it would be possible to identify costs and benefits attributable to RM, though neither could be expressed in a single unit of measurement (e.g. pounds sterling);

- the potentially broad impact of RM necessitated a detailed understanding of the processes associated with it, in order to understand how inputs (costs), processes and outcomes (benefits) were linked;

- there would be no formal controls available which would indicate what would have happened in the absence of RM;

- if the research strategy was to collect considerable amounts of new quantitative data, the data or its collection would alter the RM process itself, and in this respect the research had to be as unobtrusive as possible.

It was thus assumed that the evaluation would be broadly economic in nature, but that there were specific problems which would limit the value of such a 'black box' approach, and additional, complementary approaches would be required. These would involve a more quantitative focus on the RM process, and an examination of the way RM changed the traditional working arrangements of the hospitals.

The most important methodological problem was perceived to be the absence of formal controls for the impact of RM. In order to address this problem, the original intention was to use a 'triangulation approach' (Rossi and Freeman, 1987):

■ comparisons of specified measures before and after the management change ('reflexive' controls);

■ comparison with the 'norms' of change occurring in similar units with no formal RM intervention ('generic' controls); and

■ comparison of observed change with the judgement of the researchers, participants and others of what changes might 'ordinarily' have been expected in the pilot sites ('shadow' controls).

But as the study progressed, it became evident that the original research strategy required modification. The publication of *Working for Patients*, which led all hospitals to begin preparations for a provider market, and which announced the decision to 'roll out' RM to all large acute hospitals in the NHS, greatly increased the complexity of the task of evaluation. It represented a massive contamination of the RM 'experiment', since sites had to respond to a new agenda of issues, and compounded the problems inherent in the task of isolating the costs and benefits of RM. Further, it was realised as the research progressed, that RM was a larger and more complex phenomenon than initially realised. The result of all of these developments was to tilt the balance of the study firmly towards the qualitative. The emphasis of the work would thus be on understanding the implementation of RM and the nature of its associated management processes.

The development of this revised methodology was based on observations during the monitoring phase, that:

■ RM would not be fully implemented by the end of the study, so the research should focus on monitoring change over time, rather than on measurement after implementation was deemed to be complete;

■ costs, processes and outcomes were linked in complex ways and a part-'systems' approach was needed to elucidate the linkages between them;

■ the objectives of RM were often unclear, and indeed changed over the course of the study;

■ there were no formal controls available for RM, and the developments described above made it difficult to draw conclusions based on any other types of control;

■ it would be difficult to distinguish boundaries between RM and other hospital activities.

Underlying the last three points is the fact that the impact of RM does not conform to the experimental model, wherein it could be treated as an addition to (such as a new treatment for a condition not previously considered treatable) or a substitution for (as where a new drug treatment is introduced on the grounds that it is superior to an existing one) on-going hospital activity. RM is neither a simple addition to a hospital's activities nor just a substitution for existing ones, but a complex mixture of the two. Rather, RM is both a *cause* and a *product* of change.

The methodology adopted was based on 'modelling' the RM process. Essentially, the six pilot sites were case studies which provided the evidence, and the evaluation compares the sites against the model. Objectives, as set out in the Health Notice and as elucidated by the sites were used as benchmarks.

The methodology consisted of five steps.

1. Observing developments at the sites, treating them as case studies, over a specified period of time.

2. Identifying and clarifying *their* approaches and objectives.

3. Using the material from the sites to examine objectives and key processes.

4. Identifying the costs and benefits associated with the intervention, using a model of the process to highlight where they should be sought.

5. Evaluating the experience of the RM Initiative sites:
   (i)   against available statements of objectives;
   (ii)   against the model of the process;
   (iii) by comparing costs and benefits.

The evaluation would thus concentrate on the progress made by the sites in implementing RM against a background of major change across the NHS. It would rely to a significant extent on the experiences of participants at the sites as a basis for judgements on the success or failure of RM.

Turning to the methods used in the evaluation, these incorporated both a range of evaluative techniques and the monitoring of the RM process. The scale and complexity of RM necessitated using a variety of qualitative and quantitative methods, with work being concentrated in the six pilot sites, and within them on the chosen sub-units and clinicians. It had three components.

First, there were activities which provided evidence of the extent to which the RM process had been implemented, particularly at unit and sub-unit level, and qualitative evidence of the resource implications and value of RM. Particular aims of the work at unit and sub-unit level were to understand the similarities and differences both between, and within, sites in the implementation and operation of RM, and to obtain the judgements of participants as to the success or failure of RM. Work with sub-units was directed to an in-depth understanding of RM, and included:

- attendance at meetings, including regular 'business' meetings. Typically, these involved consultants and sub-unit managers, on a weekly or monthly basis;

- interviews with consultants, nurse managers and business managers;

- obtaining relevant documentation on sub-units' current status and plans.

This was complemented by a strategy aimed at obtaining a broad view of developments. This comprised:

- attendance at meetings. There was no meeting common to all six sites, although four of the sites held RM steering group meetings, attended by members of the Department of Health, and these were attended by the research team. Other meetings were attended on an opportunistic basis;

- interviews with specific groups across the sites, including district and unit general managers, project managers, finance managers, a range of staff responsible for computing and information handling, and 'local champions' of RM. In addition, the secretaries of the six local CHCs were interviewed, in order to obtain a more explicitly patient-oriented view of developments;

- obtaining a variety of documents relating to RM, the wider NHS reforms and the on-going business of the hospital.

The number of meetings attended and interviews conducted over the whole study is shown in Box A1.1. The totals reflect the emphasis on monitoring developments at sub-unit level. It should be stressed that the number of interviews and meetings varied between sites, reflecting the stated intention of the researchers to focus on two sites to a greater extent than the other four.

In addition, checks were made on the quality of data being collected at the sites. They were implementing major new databases, and it was thus important to check any effects on data collection. Chapter 3 reviewed the accuracy and completeness of data in the 'case mix databases' at the sites.

The second component of the work provided further evidence of the views of individuals on the costs and value of RM through two questionnaires. The first was a postal questionnaire sent to all consultants in general surgery and general medicine (including care of the elderly) in the six sites, in July 1990, with a reminder in August 1990. This achieved an 84 per cent response. The second was a questionnaire administered directly to ward sisters in the same specialties, on visits to the sites between May and July 1990.

Box A1.1   Fieldwork within the six sites 1988-90

	Meetings	*Interviews*
Sub-unit	35	75
All others	86	147
Sub-total	121	222
Total = 343		

The third component comprised quantitative evidence of activity and resource use at the sites at both sub-unit and unit levels. The financial costs of RM, and in particular the additional resources provided to the sites, were identified in discussion with the sites, although the continuing development of RM at the sites made it difficult (although important) to distinguish the investment costs involved in implementation and 'steady state' running costs of an implemented system.

Sites were asked to provide quantitative data on activity, finance and manpower, at unit and specialty levels, most of which, it was assumed, they would already be collecting as part of their national reporting requirements. It became apparent that sites would have great difficulty in providing some data (notably on manpower), and in other instances were themselves sceptical about the accuracy of their own returns. As a result, it was decided that only a subset of the requested data would be presented (see Appendix 2). It is used to illustrate general trends at the sites.

Clearly, the value of the triangulation approach was reduced by the various changes. The reflexive controls were used to measure changes over time - strictly over a specified time period rather than 'before and after' the RM intervention, but since RM was no longer the only major change affecting the sites, attributing costs and benefits to RM was made more difficult. The generic controls of what was happening in the NHS more generally were weakened because of the general endorsement of the RM approach. The shadow controls were compromised by the complexity of and uncertainty surrounding the NHS reforms, which made it very difficult to be confident of judgements about what would have happened in the absence of RM. These problems did not cause such controls to be totally abandoned, but inevitably caution was required in reaching any firm conclusions on the basis of the 'triangulation approach'.

In addition to the work at the six sites, developments at national level elsewhere in the NHS, were monitored. Principally this was achieved through obtaining relevant documentation, notably on the NHS reforms and on the 'roll-out' of RM to other hospitals. A small number of interviews with Department of Health staff were also carried out, to clarify the Department's role and perceptions of RM, both at the pilot sites and in general across the NHS.

Inevitably, the research strategy described here represents a compromise between what was theoretically desirable and what proved practicable once work commenced, and so it has both strengths and weaknesses. Taking the weaknesses of the study approach first, the problems included: the uniqueness of the individual sites, where different conclusions might have been reached from any one considered alone; the difficulties of attributing outcomes unequivocally to RM; the absence of formal controls; the confounding influence of other events, notably the NHS Review; and the fact that sites have not yet fully implemented RM, so that it is not yet possible to assess the full costs and benefits.

To set against these problems, however, there were particular strengths. These included: the depth and breadth of access to the sites, which yielded extremely rich and detailed qualitative data regarding the implementation of the RM process; the ability of a study of all six sites to illustrate diversities and commonalities of approach; and, the study's independence.

Appendix 2

TIME SERIES PERFORMANCE DATA FOR THE SIX SITES

In the future, the RM databases at the sites will undoubtedly be a rich source of research data; but by the end of 1990 they had not yet been in place long enough, and were not yet sufficiently refined to provide the necessary data on trends in service delivery across sub-units or whole units. The possibility of undertaking a limited case mix analysis, based on one or two years of data from some sites, was considered but rejected on the grounds that the time series would be too short to demonstrate substantial changes in practice, and national or regional case mix data for 1990, which might be used as a control, was not yet available.

As a result, it was decided instead to use data collected for national requirements to construct time series of key variables. The quality of this data might also be affected by the changes within the sites, but at least in principle offered the advantage of consistency of methods of data collection. In fact, the arrangements for national reporting have changed, the former Hospital Activity Analysis (HAA) returns being replaced by the Körner data set from 1987-88 onwards. The introduction of Körner brought fundamental changes in the nature of the data collected, and comparison of HAA and Körner data is fraught with problems. Accordingly, the sites were asked to supply activity, finance and manpower data only for the first three years of Körner data collection: 1987-88, 1988-89 and 1989-90. In the event, all of the sites experienced considerable difficulties in providing manpower returns, and none are presented here. Several sites had problems responding to requests for cost data, and only limited unit level data is presented here. The activity data proved less of a problem, but even here it was only readily available for all three years at unit level, and hence only unit data is presented here. Data are also presented on national trends for the same indicators as used at the sites.

Notes on tables:
N/A = not available
Accident and Emergency figures are for total new and return patients

Arrowe Park Hospital

Whole hospital activity data

	1987-88	1988-89	1989-90
Deaths and discharges:			
With day cases	40,537	40,599	40,408
Without day cases	34,094	34,300	34,516
In-patients episodes (1)			
Length of stay (days)	7.3	6.9	6.8
Turnover interval (days)	1.8	1.8	1.8
Out-patients:			
Referrals	42,161	39,745	40,372
Consultant initiated	146,022	145,633	142,568
Day cases	6,443	6,299	5,892
Accident and emergency	90,132	84,417	84,792
Ward attenders	9,102	9,643	9,617
Theatre cases	19,056	18,636	18,629
Available bed days	310,396	299,884	296,635

	£ million	£ million	£ million
Revenue budget	28.0	30.0	31.0

	£	£	£
Whole hospital costs 1989-90 prices			
In-patients:			
Per patient day	88.24	95.37	98.05
Per consultant episode	545.24	574.50	566.25
Out-patients:			
Per attendance	13.79	13.86	16.82

(1) Episodes defined as equivalent to deaths and discharges in Mersey RHA

Source: Arrowe Park Hospital

Freeman Hospital	1987-88	1988-89	1989-90
Whole hospital activity data			
Deaths and discharges:			
With day cases	36,136	N/A	N/A
Without day cases	27,705	N/A	N/A
In-patient episodes:			
With day cases	N/A	38,513	39,985
Without day cases	N/A	29,714	30,371
Length of stay (days)	7.5	6.8	5.3
Turnover interval (days)	1.8	2.5	2.2
Out-patients:			
Referrals	23,263	24,557	24,512
Consultant initiated	89,854	95,463	93,954
Day cases	8,431	8,799	9,614
Accident and emergency	881	1,633	1,815
Ward attenders	1,938	1,825	2,850
Theatre cases	24,924	25,086	26,963
Available bed days	255,751	258,962	261,836
	£ million	£ million	£ million
Revenue budget	35.6	40.0	42.1
Whole hospital costs *1989-90 prices*	£	£	£
In-patients:			
Per patient day	144.06	142.05	131.52
Per consultant/GP episode	775.19	764.38	717.86
Out-patients:			
Per attendance	28.81	31.54	33.14

Source: Freeman Hospital

Guy's Hospital

Whole hospital activity data

	1987-88	1988-89	1989-90
Deaths and discharges:			
With day cases	34,691	35,500	35,327
Without day cases	31,603	32,167	30,505
In-patient episodes:			
With day cases	N/A	N/A	36,820
Without day cases	N/A	N/A	N/A
Length of stay (days)	7.0	7.0	7.4
Turnover interval (days)	5.2	1.3	1.8
Out-patients:			
Referrals	66,412	63,433	59,452
Consultant initiated	262,033	250,997	242,925
Day cases	3,088	3,333	4,822
Accident and emergency	96,463	93,357	90,760
Ward attenders	5,418	5,662	8,939
Theatre cases	N/A	15,688	16,468
Available bed days	295,538	303,705	318,357
	£ million	*£ million*	*£ million*
Revenue budget	51.3	59.0	59.2
Whole hospital costs 1989-90 prices	*£*	*£*	*£*
In-patients:			
Per patient days	99.90	119.35	116.16
Per consultant episode	889.65	1050.42	960.99
Out-patients:			
Per attendance	30.38	47.39	28.75

Source: Guy's Hospital and South East Thames RHA

Huddersfield Royal Infirmary			
Whole hospital activity data	*1987-88*	*1988-89*	*1989-90*
Deaths and discharges:			
With day cases	N/A	N/A	N/A
Without day cases	N/A	N/A	N/A
In-patient episodes:			
With day cases	25,424	25,303	26,144
Without day cases	24,838	23,860	24,528
Length of stay (days)	5.4	5.2	5.0
Turnover interval (days)	1.7	2.0	2.4
Out-patients:			
Referrals	33,342	33,480	34,609
Consultant initiated	108,142	119,527	124,270
Day cases	586	1,443	1,616
Accident and emergency	59,972	61,726	61,949
Ward attenders	2,159	3,103	3,636
Theatre cases	10,839	12,971	12,935
Available bed days	179,823	180,156	188,867
	£ million	*£ million*	*£ million*
Revenue budget	19.1	21.0	22.0
Whole hospital costs *1989-90 prices*	*£*	*£*	*£*
In-patients:			
Per patient days			
Per consultant/GP episode	897.70	949.03	897.00
Out-patients:			
Per attendance	15.42	9.07	N/A

Source: Huddersfield Royal Infirmary

Pilgrim Hospital

Whole hospital activity data

	1987-88	*1988-89*	*1989-90*
Deaths and discharges:			
With day cases	24,476	27,101	26,389
Without day cases	22,199	24,125	24,211
In-patient episodes:			
With day cases	24,517	27,010	26,388
Without day cases	22,240	24,125	24,210
Length of stay (days)	6.8	7.0	6.8
Turnover interval (days)	2.8	3.1	3.0
Out-patients:			
Referrals	20,133	21,573	23,424
Consultant initiated	57,996	60,895	61,792
Day cases	2,277	2,885	2,178
Accident and emergency	20,263	20,300	21,235
Ward attenders	4,128	4,637	1,751
Theatre cases	10,982	11,277	11,067
Available bed days	213,716	243,520	237,408
	£ million	*£ million*	*£ million*
Revenue budget	15.3	16.6	18.3
Whole hospital costs 1989-90 prices	*£*	*£*	*£*
In-patients:			
Per patient days	72.32	119.17	115.51
Per consultant/GP episode	748.50	720.98	728.26
Out-patients:			
Per attendance	20.66	27.27	40.76

Source: Pilgrim Hospital

Royal Hampshire County Hospital			
Whole hospital activity data	*1987-88*	*1988-89*	*1989-90*
Deaths and discharges:			
With day cases	19,325	19,506	N/A
Without day cases	N/A	N/A	N/A
In-patient episodes:			
With day cases	18,817	21,114	23,678
Without day cases	17,302	19,073	20,054
Length of stay (days)	9.4	8.0	7.1
Turnover interval (days)	1.4	1.8	1.7
Out-patients:			
Referrals	20,704	20,436	23,334
Consultant initiated	66,897	66,174	68,296
Day cases	3,104	3,644	3,611
Accident and emergency	32,420	31,764	30,912
Ward attenders	1,009	4,510	3,793
Theatre cases	N/A	N/A	N/A
Available bed days	175,980	168,788	167,290
	£ million	*£ million*	*£ million*
Revenue budget	18.8	21.1	23.7
Whole hospital costs			
1989-90 prices	*£*	*£*	*£*
In-patients:			
Per patient days	89.43	101.34	89.38
Per consultant/GP episode	589.45	571.86	540.74
Out-patients:			
Per attendance	15.44	13.98	22.09
Source: Royal Hampshire County Hospital			

National trends

Acute sector
Source: NHS Hospital Activity Statistics for England
Statistical Bulletin 2/10/90
All figures except length of stay and turnover interval in thousands

	1987-88	*1988-89*	*1989-90*
Deaths and discharges:			
With day cases	N/A	N/A	N/A
Without day cases	5,061	5,009	N/A
In-patient episodes:			
With day cases	N/A	6,700	6,917
Without day cases	N/A	5,703	5,777
Length of stay (days) (1)	7.7	7.1	7.2
Turn-over interval (days)	N/A	N/A	N/A
Out-patients:			
Referrals	7,513	7,443	7,521
Consultant initiated	23,567	23,133	23,215
Day cases	860	997	1140
Accident and emergency	13,904	13,821	13,935
Ward attenders	523	579	643
Theatre cases	3,177	3,313	3,321
Available bed days (2)	128	123	121

Costs for hospital units
Source: CIPFA 1990 Health Database. Figures based on returns from
approximately two-thirds of Health Authorities in England and Wales

	£	£	£
In-patients:			
Per patient day	N/A	126.54	114.50
Per consultant episode	N/A	650.87	724.20
Out-patients:			
Per attendance	N/A	29.50	29.30

1 = crude average for medicine and surgery only. 1989-90 figures from
CIPFA 1990 Health Database
2 = average for acute sector

GLOSSARY

■ *Business manager.* A staff member who works in a sub-unit of a hospital, such as a clinical specialty, a directorate or a department. The business manager assists the head (who is normally a practising professional) with aspects of management of the sub-unit; particularly collecting and interpreting information, planning and monitoring performance.

■ *Case mix classification systems.* Methods for assigning numerical or alphabetical/ numerical codes to procedures and diagnoses, to facilitate analysis of patient treatment. Classification systems are typically ordered by organ system.

■ *Clinical directorate.* Sub-unit organisation structure, based on a defined group of patient services, such as general surgery or pathology, that is devolved responsibility for the management of its own activities. It is multi-disciplinary, and managed by a director who is usually a clinician.

■ *Coding.* Translating medical diagnoses and procedures into a numerical or alphabetical/numerical classification that can be used for purposes of recording activity and statistical analysis.

■ *Diagnosis Related Groups (DRGs).* A method of classifying inpatients into groups based upon coherent clinical application and homogeneous use of resources. There are currently some 500 DRGs in the version used most widely in the USA.

■ *General management.* Responsibility for the overall performance and development of the particular entity, such as a service, a hospital, a health district or a health region, being managed. The basic level of general management in the NHS is the unit, which may comprise a hospital, or hospitals, a territory, a service or group of related services.

■ *Griffiths recommendations.* A Committee chaired by (Sir) Roy Griffiths, which investigated the management of the NHS, reporting in 1983. Among their recommendations were the implementation of general management, an increased involvement in management by service providers and more attention to commercial principles.

■ *Hospital Information System (HIS).* An operational computer system linking wards and departments which has facilities for ordering and reporting.

■ *ICD-9-CM.* The International Classification of Diseases, 9th edition, Clinical Modification.

- *Körner data sets.* The data collected by hospitals and community health services for reporting to the Department of Health, as specified by the Körner Steering Committee on Health Services Information, 1982-1984.

- *Management Budgeting (MB).* An experiment, developed by the Griffiths Inquiry, to try and involve service providers in determining, managing and monitoring their budgets. The predecessor of RM.

- *Medical audit.* The NHS Review obliged all doctors to engage in audit (although many already did so) examining the quality of their care collectively with other members of their specialty, clinical group or practice. Primarily an educational tool, audit also has implications for service management; general managers must be informed of overall results and can initiate specific audits.

- *NHS Review.* Undertaken by senior members of the Conservative Government and their advisers during 1988. The results, published as a White Paper *Working for Patients* in early 1989, and translated into law by the National Health Service and Community Care Act, 1990, represent a fundamental change to both the principles of the NHS and its organisation.

- *Opportunity costs.* Because resources are limited, when they are applied to one particular object, such as RM, other objects to which the resources might have been applied may suffer. So development for one object represents opportunity costs for others.

- *Patient Administration System (PAS).* A computerised information system which typically contains basic information about patients, such as name, address and date of birth, and details of their admission and discharge from hospital.

- *Read clinical classification.* A classification system for use in coding procedures, diagnoses, signs and symptoms into alphabetical and numerical form. It was developed by James Read, a GP based in Loughborough, UK, and adopted by the Department of Health for use by GPs in recording their activity.

- *RM database.* The principal database management system implemented by the RM pilot sites. A centralised database designed to support planning, monitoring and evaluation of patient services.

- *Resource Management (RM) Initiative.* The RM Initiative was introduced as a national experiment in six pilot acute hospital sites in 1986. A provisional evaluation was undertaken in 1988 and a further evaluation in 1989. By then, RM had become NHS policy.

- *Service activity benefits*. Improvements to the patient services that are provided, such as reduced waiting time or quicker referrals.

- *Service production benefits*. Improvements to the way in which patient services are organised, such as faster and more accurate communications or improved use of staff.

- *Service providers*. Those staff, such as doctors, nurses, paramedical, scientific, some managers and some ancillary staff, whose work is directly concerned with giving diagnostic, treatment, caring or counselling services to patients.

- *Specialty division*. The grouping together of medical staff in related areas of work for representative, advisory, managerial and/or audit purposes. Different groupings may be required for different purposes but a common example would be the Orthopaedic Division or General Surgical Division.

- *Sub-unit*. Hospital units may be divided up into sub-units with devolved authority, such as departments and/or directorates. Some sub-unit organisation is traditional but it has been fragmented. Directorates introduce a level of sub-unit organisation across the whole unit.

- *Unit*. Health districts are subdivided into units, each with their own general manager. Units may comprise a hospital, hospitals, a territory, a service or group of related services. The RM Initiative was directed to six acute hospital units.

- *User group*. A collection of staff who are all working with a particular RM facility, such as an information system. The group may be disciplinary, such as a clinical or nursing user group, or multi-disciplinary, representing a directorate. User groups provide a valuable means of liaison with RM project staff.

REFERENCES

Alford, R. (1975). *Health Care Politics*. Chicago, University of Chicago Press.

Association of Community Health Councils for England and Wales (1990). *RMI - Resource Management Initiative or Rushed, Mismanaged and Inept?* London, ACHCEW.

Bagust, A. (1989). Resource Management or Managing Resources?, *Health Services Management Research*, **2**, (3), 217-20.

Bardsley, M., Coles, J. and Jenkins, L. (eds), (1987). *DRGs in Health Care*. (2nd edition). London, King Edward's Hospital Fund.

Black, A., Dearden, B., Mathew, D. and Nichol, D. (1989). *The Extension of Resource Management: An Audit for Action*. Bristol, NHS Training Authority.

Brooks, A.P. (1990). Clinical directorates, *British Medical Journal*, **300**, 1141.

Burns, T. and Stalker, G. (1966). *The Management of Innovation*. London, Social Science Paperbacks.

Buxton, M., Packwood, T. and Keen, J. (1989). *Resource Management: Process and Progress*. Uxbridge, Brunel University.

Buxton, M., Packwood, T. and Keen, J. (1991). *Final Report of the Brunel University Evaluation of Resource Management*. Uxbridge, Brunel University.

Central Consultants and Specialists Committee (1989). *An Evaluation of the Six Experimental Sites by the CCSC*. London, British Medical Association.

Chantler, C. (1989). How to do it: Be a Manager, *British Medical Journal*, **298**, 1505-08.

Checkland, P.B. (1988). Information Systems and Systems Thinking: Time to Unite?, *International Journal of Information Management*, **8**, 239-48.

Coffey, R.M. (1980). *How a Medical Information System Affects Hospital Costs: The El Camino Hospital Experience*. Washington DC, US Department of Health, Education and Welfare, National Center for Health Services Research.

Coles, J., Davison, A. and Wickings, I. (1974). Control of Resources, *Health and Social Service Journal*, 16 November, 2654-5.

Coles, J., Davison, A. and Wickings, I. (1976). Allocating Budgets to Wards: an Experiment, *The Hospital and Health Services Review*, September, 309-12.

Committee of Public Accounts (1990). *Financial Management in the National Health Service*. Sixteenth Report. London, HMSO.

Coombs, R., Knights, D. and Willmott, H. (1990). *Culture, Control and Competitiveness: Towards a Conceptual Framework for the Study of Information Technology in Organisations*. CROMTEC Working Paper 3, Manchester School of Management, UMIST.

Coombs, R., Bloomfield, B. and Rea, D. (1991). Differences in a Scheme of Change. *Health Service Journal*, 24 January, 16.

Department of Health (1989a). RM: The Guy's Story. (Video).

Department of Health (1989b). RM: The Nurses' View. (Video).

Department of Health (1989c). *Project Planning*. London, Department of Health.

Department of Health (1990a). NHS Hospital Activity Statistics for England, 1979-1989/90, Bulletin 2/10/90. London, Department of Health.

Department of Health (1990b). *Nursing Information Requirements*. London, Department of Health.

DHSS (1982-84). Steering Group on Health Services Information. (Körner Reports). London, Department of Health and Social Security.

DHSS (1985). Health Service Management. Management Budgeting, Health Notice HN(85)3. London, Department of Health and Social Security.

DHSS (1986a). Health Services Management - Resource Management (Management Budgeting) in Health Authorities, Health Notice, HN(86)34. London, Department of Health and Social Security.

DHSS (1986b). *A National Strategic Framework for Information Management in the Hospital and Community Health Services*. London, Department of Health and Social Security.

DHSS (1988). Method for Identifying the Costs and Benefits of Computer Systems used in Health Care, *Information Management in the Hospital and Community Health Services*. London, DHSS IT Division.

Disken, S., Dixon, M., Halpern, S. and Shocket, G. (1990). *Models of Clinical Management*. London, Institute of Health Services Management.

Ernst and Young Management Consultants (1990). *Information systems services: Aligning business, people and IT*. London, Ernst and Young.

Eyles, J. (1987). *The Geography of the National Health*. London, Croom Helm.

Fuchs, V. (1974). *Who Shall Live?* New York, Basic Books.

Galliers, R. (ed.) (1987). *Information Analysis*. Sydney, Addison Wesley.

Griffiths, R. (1983). NHS Management Inquiry, *(The Griffiths Report)*, London, Department of Health and Social Security.

Griffiths, R. (1988). *An Agenda for Action*, London, HMSO.

Ham, C. (1986). *Managing Health Services*, SAUS Study No 3. School of Advanced Urban Studies, University of Bristol.

Ham, C. and Hunter, D. (1988). *Managing Clinical Activity in the NHS*. London, King's Fund Institute.

Henderson, J.C. and Venkatraman, N. (1989). *Strategic Alignment: A Process Model for Integrating Information Technology and Business Strategies*, Sloan School of Management, 77 Massachusetts Avenue, Cambridge, Massachusetts, 02193: Centre for Information Systems Research, Massachusetts Institute of Technology.

HM Treasury (1991). *Public Expenditure Analyses to 1993-94*. Cmnd 1520. London, HMSO.

Institute of Health Services Managers/National Association of Health Authorities (1989). *Income Generation in the NHS*. London, King's Fund Institute.

Keen, H. (1990). Clinical directorates. Letter to *British Medical Journal*, 300, 945.

Klein, R. (1989). *The Politics of the NHS*. (2nd edition) London, Longman.

Masters, S. (1990). A Natural Evolution, *Health Service Journal*, 12 April, 555.

Millar, B. (1987). Resource Management Pilot Sites on Air. *Health Service Journal*, 29 October, 1250.

National Audit Office (1990). *Managing Computer Projects in the NHS*. London, HMSO.

NHS Management Executive (1990). *Financial Management Update*. Issue 2. London, NHS Finance Directorate.

NHS Training Authority (1990). *Guide to the Implementation of Nursing Information Systems*, Bristol, NHSTA.

NHS Resource Management Unit (1990). *Resource Management: The Leading Edge*. London, NHS Finance Directorate.

Oxford Regional Health Authority (1988). *Management Budgeting Evaluation Report: The Radcliffe Infirmary, Oxford*. Oxford, Oxford Regional Health Authority.

Packwood, T., Buxton, M. and Keen, J. (1990). Resource Management in the National Health Service, *Policy and Politics*, **18**, (4), 245-55.

Perrin, J. (1988). *Resource Management in the NHS*. Wokingham, Van Nostrand Reinhold.

Pollitt, C., Harrison, S., Hunter, D. and Marnoch, G. (1988). The reluctant managers: clinicians and budgets in the NHS. *Financial Accountability and Management*, **4**, 213-33.

Prowle, M., Jones, T. and Shaw, J. (1989). *Working for Patients: The Financial Agenda*. London, Chartered Association of Certified Accountants.

RM Directorate (1989). *Resource Management Initiative: Information Package - Acute Hospitals*. London, Department of Health.

Rossi, P.H. and Freeman, H.E. (1987). *Evaluation: A Systematic Approach*. (3rd edition). Beverley Hills (CA), Sage.

Rowen, R.B. (1990). Software Project Management Under Incomplete and Ambiguous Specifications. *IEEE Transactions on Engineering Management*, **37**, 10-21.

Royal College of General Practitioners (1989). *The Classification and Analysis of General Practice Data*. Occasional Paper 26, (2nd edition) London, RCGP.

Secretaries of State for Health, Scotland, Wales and Northern Ireland (1987). *Promoting Better Health*, Cmnd 248. London, HMSO.

Secretaries of State for Health, Scotland, Wales and Northern Ireland (1989a). *Working for Patients*. Cmnd 555. London, HMSO.

Secretaries of State for Health, Social Security, Wales and Scotland (1989b). *Caring for People*. Cmnd 849. London, HMSO.

Smith, N. and Chantler, C. (1987). Partnership for Progress. *Public Finance and Accountancy*, May, 12-14.

Social Services Committee of the House of Commons (1989). Eighth Report, *Resourcing the National Health Service: The Government's Plans for the Future of the National Health Service*. London, HMSO.